Neighborhood Networks for Humane Mental Health Care

Neighborhood Networks for Humane Mental Health Care

Arthur J. Naparstek

University of Southern California
Washington Public Affairs Center
Washington, D.C.

David E. Biegel

School of Social Work
University of Pittsburgh
Pittsburgh, Pennsylvania

and

Herzl R. Spiro

Distinguished Professor of Research Psychiatry
Medical College of Wisconsin
Milwaukee, W.I.

with Joseph Coffey and John Andreozzi

PLENUM PRESS • NEW YORK AND LONDON

Library of Congress Cataloging in Publication Data

Main entry under title:

Neighborhood networks for humane mental health care.

Includes bibliographical references and index.
1. Community mental health services—United States. 2. Community psychology. I.
Naparstek, Arthur. II. Biegel, David E. III. Spiro, Herzl R., 1935–   . [DNLM: 1.
Community mental health services—Organization and Administration—United
States. WM 30 N3966]
RA790.6.N44 1982   362.2′0425   82-18149
ISBN 0-306-41051-6

©1982 Plenum Press, New York
A Division of Plenum Publishing Corporation
233 Spring Street, New York, N.Y. 10013

Printed in the United States of America

To Msgr. Geno Baroni
who exemplifies what the Judeo-Christian ethic is all about.
His capacity for vision in a troubled and cynical world is rare.
Father Baroni's belief in our work gave birth to this book;
and to the residents of
South East Baltimore City and the Southside, City of Milwaukee.
It was their cooperation that made the book an actuality.

Foreword

It is hard to think of a more timely and topical major contribution than Drs. Naparstek, Biegel, Spiro, and collaborators have provided in this volume. Their penetrating, comprehensive study and field tests give us mapping toward the goal of reifying the concept of "community" as applied to human services. The book will prove invaluable to those at the policy level—legislators, planners, and administrators. It will serve as an essential reference for community workers—professional providers, natural helpers, and citizens as a whole.

A salient ideal of New Federalism—placing governance as close to the people as practicable—seems a prophetic match with the model of Neighborhood Empowerment. As the authors point out, conventional wisdom has seemed to offer government regulation, control, and program evaluation as a panacea package for improving human services. This work suggests a radically different approach; specifically, a shift to greater instrumental involvement of the richly variegated mosaic of American neighborhoods, combined with a system of excellent, high technology service agencies.

Certainly, genuine efforts have been made before toward a true linkage of the community with human services. The Great Society programs, with their emphasis on citizen involvement and "maximum feasible participation" established the foundation for legitimate citizen/consumer linkage with the program process.

Yet, in so many instances, the results fell far short of expectations. Citizens were invited to gather for reviewing and advising on annual program evaluation reports. But few appeared. When groups of citizens mobilized action they sometimes represented special interest factions rather than the population of the total community. Consumer advocacy efforts too often turned out to be adversarial, occasionally impairing subsequent service delivery. It became clear that calling a group of area residents a "community board" did not transform a facility into a community-directed entity with capacity to help people when and where they needed it.

There are, of course, numerous examples of successful community linkage in certain program focuses. Crime prevention, commercial and economic revitalization, and housing services represent issues around which community citizens and institutions participate in established program operations. Community mental health services are not without some successes in this regard. But for the most part, effective mutual participation has proved to be a difficult process to bring about. Perhaps the stigma of mental problems has deterred some persons. To many, mental health no longer strikes them as sufficiently vivid and exciting to warrant an investment of efforts. Further, there are few visible rewards, such as gaining a needed traffic light might provide.

In the Community Mental Health Empowerment Model, the authors clearly have demonstrated that the barriers indeed can be overcome. *Empowerment* does not mean that communities "take over." Mutual participation is the keystone. It strives for symmetry—the alignment of public servants and citizens and the development of a sense of empathy between them. The Model recognizes that professionals, operating within their professional capacities, are entitled to appropriate status, dignity, and respect. And similarly, neighborhood leaders, natural helpers, and members of other mediating structures (such as the church) are entitled to meet with health professionals on a level of comparable status, dignity, and respect.

The Model emphasizes the unique strengths of city neighborhoods so that support systems are mobilized. Networks are created to link professional and informal service systems. The objective is to identify and overcome obstacles which prevent community residents from seeking and receiving help. In achieving this objective, the Model is intended to help people gain a sense of control over their lives, reduce alienation from society, acquire the capacity to solve new problems, and to sustain motivation to overcome the handicaps and frustrations which are common to modern society.

One can hardly question that such an approach is sorely needed to further help community mental health become in actuality what the concept implies. But does it work? Are there benefits? The answers to both have to be resounding affirmatives.

The authors furnish cogent evidence that through the neighborhood support systems approach inherent in the Model populations can indeed be reached who are in need of assistance but unwilling or unable to seek professional help. The community's sense of competency and worth are increased because the approach builds upon strengths rather than weaknesses and enhances the neighborhood's pre-existing systems of informal support. Consumer involvement is enriched and agencies become more effectively accountable at the neighborhood level. The linkages that necessarily develop between mental health and other human service programs reduce fragmentation and needless costs.

The Community Mental Health Empowerment Model is not an innovation that can be implemented by quick and easy steps. The authors are clear in pointing out that they offer no simple blueprint. The process is time-consuming and yields slow results. I would strongly advise consultative assistance in reaching a decision on adopting the model in a given setting. Consultation at points throughout the implementation also is advisable toward attaining the full potential yield of this promising and needed approach.

This book provides a superb learning opportunity in community aspects of community mental health, in addition to serving as an exciting introduction and guide to this pivotal model.

The authors are extraordinarily qualified for this work as scholars, scientists, and practitioners; further, their sound lessons learned from direct experiences of the Sixties are evident throughout this volume. We owe them deep gratitude for this outstanding contribution to community mental health.

HOWARD R. DAVIS

Chief, Mental Health Services
Research and Development Branch National Institutes of Mental
Health
Rockville, Maryland

Acknowledgments

This book is an outgrowth of the Neighborhood and Family Services Project, a four-year research and demonstration effort funded by grant #R01MH2653 from the Mental Health Services Development Branch, National Institute of Mental Health, to the University of Southern California, Washington Public Affairs Center. There are many groups and individuals that greatly aided our work. We owe a special debt of gratitude to Dr. Howard R. Davis, Chief, Mental Health Services Development Branch, National Institute of Mental Health, whose interest, support, and enthusiasm assisted us immeasurably. Special thanks are also given to Msgr. Geno Baroni, under whose leadership the project was sponsored in the first grant year at the National Center for Urban Ethnic Affairs.

The residents of South East Baltimore and the Southside of Milwaukee with whom we worked, unselfishly devoted themselves to planning, organizing, developing programs, raising monies, and in general helping to prove that neighborhood empowerment can work. Their dedication, zeal, and competence made a tremendous contribution to the project's success. We probably learned as much from them as they did from us.

This book would not have been possible without the support and encouragement of our respective schools. We therefore thank the University of Southern California, School of Public Administration; the University of Pittsburgh, School of Social Work; and the Medical College of Wisconsin for allowing us the time to complete this volume.

Joseph Coffey and John Andreozzi, field coordinators in Baltimore and Milwaukee, respectively, throughout the course of the entire four-year period assumed the major responsibility for implementing project activities on the local level. In the preparation of this manuscript they wrote the initial drafts of Chapters 9 and 10, respectively, while also contributing some material that was utilized in other parts of the book.

Mohammad Khan served as Research Director of the project and assisted in the field research for this volume. Elsa Solendar provided invaluable assistance in the preparation and organization of the manuscript, while Linda Wykoff is thanked for her efficient and accurate typing and editing of the text. Without Leah Gansler's involvement with the final draft, this volume would not have been completed. The authors owe her a great deal. Karen Klein, Wendy Sherman, and Barbara Spence served as project staff members in varying capacities and made significant contributions. Any errors of fact or interpretation remain, of course, the responsibility of the authors.

ARTHUR J. NAPARSTEK
DAVID E. BIEGEL
HERZL R. SPIRO

Contents

PART ONE

CHAPTER 1

In Search of a Human Scale

Future decades may chronicle the failure of a vast network of "community" mental health programs in the United States that never really existed. The landmark Community Mental Health Centers Act of 1963 sought the transfer of principal responsibility for treating mental illness and promoting mental health from state mental hospitals to a network of mental health centers in places called "the community." By 1980, a mere 800 of the 2,000 community mental health centers (CMHCs) envisioned in the 1963 act actually existed. Yet the policy of "deinstitutionalizing" patients from state hospitals to the "community" continued, even where community care was totally absent. Of the 800 CMHCs, few had much to do with "community."

This book is about two of the exceptions: two city neighborhoods where community mental health and human service programs not only exist but actually work. It attempts to describe how and why they work, and ways in which they may serve as models for other communities elsewhere. The practical programs described here developed as a result of the authors' recognition of two misconceptions that have, unfortunately, characterized the development—and the lack of development—of the community mental health movement. As should now be evident to all serious analysts:

- Slapping a sign that reads "Community Mental Health Center" onto a storefront does not create a community.
- Calling a group of area residents a "Board of Directors" does not transform a federally mandated institution into a community-directed entity with the capacity to help people where and when they need help.

We have not proceeded on the assumption that a mental health center in a community is a bad idea. But we have observed that even where community mental health centers do in fact exist *in* communities, they rarely are part *of* their communities.

We believe that effective community mental health programs need

3

to be conceived and operated on a genuinely human scale. We believe in the empowerment of people in their neighborhoods so that they themselves may develop and direct appropriate service systems relevant to their own needs. We believe that working partnerships need to be created between empowered neighborhoods and mental health institutions. Implicit in our approach is a full appreciation of the meaning of such widely used—and misused—terms as *community, neighborhood, mental health, alienation,* and *empowerment.* In the process of elucidating our understanding of these concepts, we intend to suggest the significance and scope of the term *human scale* as we understand it.

This book introduces our conception of practical mental health services on a human scale. It suggests some of the major problems that have hindered the development of such systems in American cities. In describing the community mental health movement as it seems to us to be today, our plan is to suggest how it ought to be—and can be—in the future.

THE ACUTELY ILL AND THE "WORRIED WELL": WHO SHALL BE SERVED AND WHERE?

One recurring problem in developing an effective approach to community mental health has been the difficulty of distinguishing populations to be served by the mental health care system. In some places, there has been little distinction between neighborhood mental health and the wholesale dumping of chronic psychotics from state hospitals into boarding houses. Proponents of such immoral dumping justify themselves by singing the praises of "delabeling" and "deinstitutionalization." Little wonder that many neighborhoods want nothing to do with community mental health. In other places, neighborhood mental health has stood for ignoring the severely ill and delivering the old wine of traditional social services to all families in new bottles labeled "community mental health." Such slick packaging offers little in the way of practical support for the severely ill, who are once more consigned to chronic institutions: prisons, ill-equipped nursing homes, board-and-care houses, and state hospitals. A tension has emerged between those who define community mental health services in terms of the preventive and supportive functions that neighborhoods do best, and those who define the problem exclusively as care for the most severely ill. One way of resolving this tension will be to define more specifically who shall be served and at which locus of care.

Mental health services must focus on at least two overlapping groups of people. One group needs assistance with the problems, stresses, and crises of everyday life that produce the symptoms and behavior of the "worried well." Their day-to-day problems of loneliness, sadness, tension, marital discord, and family stress do not fit neatly into discrete categories. Definition in terms of individual dysfunction may need to give way to redefinition in terms of environmental and community dysfunction. Self-help mechanisms that already exist in a neighborhood, or might be developed through the neighborhood environment, may be most useful to this population. Professional services should certainly play a supportive role, but they ought to be designed to enhance, not replace, neighborhood empowerment.[1] Careful analysis will reveal, however, that there will never be, nor should there be, a sufficient critical mass of high-technology professional services to meet all of the problems of the "worried well." The professional can and should serve as consultant in the provision of services for this group,but the primary providers of care must be by neighbor-

---

[1]Definition of empowerment: *Empowerment* is a term that may be defined from a host of different perspectives. Two concepts provide a framework for the way in which the term is utilized in this volume: capacity and equity. Capacity may be defined in three ways: (a) It is an individual's or group's ability to utilize power to solve problems; (b) it is a group's or individual's ability to gain access to institutions or organizations that are serving them; and (c) it is an individual's or group's ability to nurture and accommodate. Power and nurturance depend on different types of resources. Power involves skills and financial resources. The skills required for the effective exercise of power include organization, leadership, management, and the technical expertise to plan, conduct research, and implement projects. Financial resources for power include money, capital, and other assets needed for skill development and project implementation. The defining elements of the nurturance dimension of capacity are human and community resources. Included here are people expressing themselves through family, through neighboring, and through voluntary networks such as churches, PTAs, ethnic groups, fraternal associations, veterans' organizations, taverns, soda fountains, and street corners. These are contexts that bond people together, develop support systems, and form a personal basis for living. Human and community resources exist to some degree in every neighborhood. They are natural resources of the neighborhoods. In turn, neighborhoods are natural resources of cities, with unique reserves of personal commitment to others, of volunteer energy ready to be tapped and channeled. The other forms of capacity are the necessary means of tapping such resources. Each neighborhood is unique, so each requires a different mix of skills and financial resources (National Commission on Neighborhoods, 1979b). *Equity:* The principle of equity is defined by citizens in two ways: whether their investment (objective or subjective) is equal to their return; and whether their neighborhood organization is getting its fair share of resources as compared to other parts of the city. Thus, when citizens invest through the tax system, they expect a return in services and amenities. However, the problem is complicated in that the return is not within the complete control of the citizens or even of local decision makers (Naparstek & Haskell, 1977).

hood-based support systems[2] because of what must be recognized as insurmountable economic barriers to the provision of high-quality professional care for everyone.

A second group requiring service consists primarily of desperately ill people who experience phenomena such as overpowering depression, suicidal impulses, loss of contact with reality, major disorders of thought, severe delusions, flagrant hallucinations, catatonic excitement, and so forth. These are signs and symptoms of severe psychiatric illness, which in turn fit three functional subgroups. Some of these patients experience a single episode and recover. Others experience multiple episodes but are not severely impaired between illnesses. A third small subgroup remains severely ill and needs a long-term safe haven. When patients with high symptom levels are dropped into neighborhood boarding houses and halfway houses without adequate treatment systems, neighborhood residents are likely to stigmatize and reject them, both as specific individuals and as part of the general population of the mentally ill. This process of negative attitude formation may adversely affect the "worried well." The very small group of chronic severely ill patients needs help in havens outside the neighborhood. Until this is fully acknowledged, both the acute treatment hospitals, with their high costs, and the potential neighborhood support systems will be misdirected and overwhelmed by what is really a very small minority of patients. Acute severely ill individuals require high-technology interventions by skilled professionals. If mental health institutions could be linked to empowered neighborhood structures, the rehabilitation phase for those who are not impaired severely or chronically could be more readily accomplished. Neighborhood placement would become more viable, particularly for those who experience long periods of merely mild impairment or even the absence of dysfunction between attacks. Potentially curable, the episodic illnesses would not be turned into iatrogenic social breakdown syndromes.

Confusing the various groups of patients that have been described can only lead to mischief. Neighborhood problems can best be handled in the neighborhood. When the "worried well" are institutionalized, costs mount up, day-to-day problems are mislabeled, and people are deprived of needed family and neighborhood support structures. When the severely ill are made the burden of emerging neighborhood structures, discouragement and disillusion set in. Much of the problem of the delivery of mental health service in the 1960s and 1970s may have

---

[2]Family, friends, neighbors, clergy, ethnic organizations, self-help groups, neighborhood organizations, and so forth.

been caused by the wrong people being sent to the wrong places for care. An entrenched government bureaucracy and self-serving politicians have compounded this problem in the interest of perpetuating their jobs and power in the status quo.

In any given year, at least 15% of the population shows symptoms of such severity as to be considered mentally ill (President's Commission on Mental Health, 1978). If mild or moderate anxieties and emotional upsets are included, the percentages are much higher; 15% is thus a conservative minimum rate. If all of the available professional mental health resources were maximally deployed, no more than 3% of the population could receive professional care at any given time. Many of the 3% who could be treated in the formal mental health system could not receive high-technology intervention, given current professional shortages. They would be seen by insufficiently trained mental health assistants and would receive what amounts to "Band-Aid" care. If only 3% of the population can be treated in the mental health care system in any given year, what is to become of the remaining 12% whose symptoms are severe enough to warrant a diagnosis of major psychiatric illness? What of the additional millions who exhibit symptoms but do not fit into rigid criteria of major mental illness? The President's Commission on Mental Health (1978) commends these patients to the care of "community support systems." What community support systems? What is a community support system? How can it evolve? What does it include? Is there enough support for the "worried well" as well as the moderately ill persons for whom direct professional services may not be available? Reassessment of available services and priorities is critically needed; so is the redefinition of neighborhood support and service systems.

This volume is not intended to provide models for high-technology interventions with the acute severely ill and the chronic severely impaired. This omission does not represent failure to appreciate the importance of such programs. We hope we have made neither the error of preaching that the neighborhood is sufficient unto itself nor the error, "Leave it to the massive government hospital." If neighborhoods are to link with hospitals and medical facilities, these too must be designed as human scale institutions with "docking mechanisms" for neighborhood access and egress. However, the purpose of this book is to describe the missing neighborhood side of the system. A separate volume is in preparation to describe such high-technology institutions and interventions. Neither volume would be sufficient unto itself.

CHAPTER 2

The Need for a Micromodel

Mental health and human services are being reassessed once again today. But the purpose of these studies is in good part misdirected. Analysts are attempting to define issues in a period of economic scarcity. Distribution of services has historically tended to follow the dollar. Consequently, major emphasis has been placed on such matters as financial accountability, cost effectiveness, and efficiency. These are salient "dollar issues," which one must not lose sight of, but such fiscal exercises offer no *service* insights.

Money, or cost saving, is not and should not be the prime rationale for alterations in the ways in which services are delivered. Such money saving often proves itself uneconomical. Gutted programs are sometimes worse than no programs. Model building must be based on people's needs. The discontent and discomfort of America's urban populace is not related solely to quantifiable matters such as the cost of services or fee-for-service rates. We believe that a profound alienation pervades our urban populace, encompassing feelings of powerlessness, meaninglessness, isolation, and self-estrangement. The underlying challenge is to ascertain whether the roots of alienation can be found in the neighborhood, and whether human services in a neighborhood can make a difference in reversing or expurgating those elements of community life that alienate. The tendency to define a situation and objectives in dollar terms has not resulted in the creation of effective models to improve services. Where might such models be found?

Rather than search for new program and administrative models, a whole new approach seems to be required for us to avoid the pitfalls of the past. During the past two decades, most human problems have been defined in the context of macrosocial and economic forces. The persistent failure of programs designed by governments to be directly relevant to the needs of people can be traced to the policy makers' insistence on diagnosing and prescribing for all ills on the grand scale almost exclusively. The assumptions and beliefs underlying the service initiatives and theoretical systems of the 1960s and 1970s were not directed towards the microaspects of problem solving in a neighborhood context. Virtually all efforts to halt the decline of our cities have been marked by a failure to define national policy on a human scale. Therefore, policy makers have not developed policy initiatives that serve the varied needs of differing neighborhoods. If we are to speak realistically of preconditions required for effective changes, it must be recognized that the neighborhood—not the sprawling, anonymous megalopolis—is the key. In real terms, people's investments—emotional as well as economic—are in neighborhoods, not cities. The city cannot survive if its neighborhoods continue to decline.

We propose a new analysis of the potential of a neighborhood approach in policy and programmatic terms. We recognize that any model for a neighborhood approach ought to fulfill four general prerequisites. First and foremost, involvement of all concerned sectors in a city is required. Second, the approach must be pluralistic to be successful, cognizant of the diverse needs of different groups of people. Third, the need for "appropriate scaling" is crucial. This is not a question of absolute size, but of determining the appropriate scale for what we are trying to do. Some activities are best undertaken on a large scale. In Schumacher's words, "for his purposes, man needs many different structures, both small ones and large ones, some exclusive and some comprehensive" (Schumacher, 1973). Fourth, the objective of neighborhood efforts—to aid specific individuals who have specific needs—must never be overlooked. Neighborhoods can be expected neither to perform appendectomies nor to treat catatonic excitement. Neighborhood engagement must be on a level that permits effective programs, not doctor-for-a-day fantasies!

Mental health programs have often been "parachuted" into communities. They are operated with few, if any, ties to the neighborhood-based organizational and cultural support systems. A full understanding of the intercultural dimensions of neighborhood life, particularly in relation to service delivery, has not yet evolved. A consequence is that the inherent strengths of ethnic groups have not been utilized in identifying cases, or in prevention or rehabilitation programs. The problem is made more complex because of our insufficient understanding of the interdependence among race, ethnicity, social class, and well-being.

For mental health programs to achieve a truly human scale, several major departures from current "conventional wisdom" seem to be required. The authors seriously doubt that federal, state, or local government can operate any programs on a truly human scale, whether they are programs for neighborhoods or for high-technology care.

Direct government interventions—so popular in the 1960s—often destroyed what they were intended to support. Governments do not create neighborhoods. Neighborhoods grow upward from people, not downward from programs. Governments cannot even seem to operate high-technology hospitals without creating more problems than they solve. The desirability of judicious infusions of financial resources and meaningful regulation must no longer be confused with direct interference by government agencies in the delivery of care. If the past two decades have taught us anything, it should have been the limitations of direct government operations (Spiro, 1980a). The heavy hand of direct government operation must be removed from both hospitals and neighborhood efforts.

THE NEIGHBORHOOD AS CONTEXT FOR CARE

The efficacy of a mental health delivery system depends largely on recognizing the proper context for delivery of care. There is a context for treating severe disease, and there is a context for building community support structures. Despite much rhetoric about supporting community involvement, psychiatrists, psychologists, and social workers have shown little real understanding of the dynamics of urban life. Many mental health planners have behaved as if social agencies or community mental health centers are the community. Federal mental health planners usually define a community as some unit of government. But the average working person knows that his "community" is not a government but a neighborhood.

Neighborhoods, like people, have distinct personalities. Middle-class Italian neighborhoods in Baltimore deal with problems differently from Jewish neighborhoods in Chicago, whose residents in turn face crises and seek help differently from Hispanic, black, Polish, or Irish neighborhoods elsewhere. Yet planners of government programs have usually acted as if American urban communities were uniform building blocks, waiting to be fit into some enormous superstructure with the "Made in Washington" or "Made in the State House" label—a label that many people with emotional and economic investments in city neighborhoods have learned to distrust from painful experiences.

The tendency has been to diagnose and prescribe for mental health problems exclusively on the grand scale, not on the human scale. We have failed to capitalize on the strengths of neighborhoods that have existing resources. In fact, we have undermined many community-based initiatives. Neighborhood-based approaches to meeting the needs of people can be critical to individual well-being (President's Commission on Mental Health, 1978, p. 159). R. Warren notes that strengthening neighborhood networks can help people: (a) gain a sense of control over their lives; (b) reduce alienation from society; (c) acquire capacity to solve new problems; and (d) sustain the motivation to overcome the handicaps and frustrations that are common to modern society (President's Commission on Mental Health, 1978, p. 159).

The concept of decentralization of service delivery systems in neighborhoods has arisen in response to a number of ill-defined and interwoven pressures and forces, some of them endemic to the cultural atmosphere in our cities, some at work in federal and municipal governments themselves. A major factor is the perception of a general lack of effectiveness of existing centralized service delivery systems, an appearance that all too often accurately reflects reality. The failure of urban service delivery bureaucracies to meet the needs of their neighborhood clientele derives largely from the trend to centralize that, until recently, has marked most public administration and governmental reform movements in this country. Paradoxically, centralization, which invariably translates into power acquistion by government, civil-service bureaucrats, is often introduced "to save money," but more often than not it costs money. Not only has centralization of bureaucracies led to application of uniform systematic approaches to unique neighborhood problems, where flexible, diversified approaches would have been more appropriate to the objectives, but it has also resulted in a concomitant overbureaucratization—additional layers of administrators to separate the clientele from the services they seek. Effective reform will be impossible until an effective counterforce is found to these self-serving, administrator bureaucracies, which are composed of people with ample time, motive, and skill to lobby and delude well-meaning, elected officials. The idealistic, task-oriented administrator is too often overwhelmed by hordes of civil-service bureaucrats defending their jobs and perquisites.

Over the last decade, we have seen a sharp rise in demand for a wide range of human services, as well as the simpler sorts of traditional physical services. Delivery of human services poses numerous difficulties. Kahn and others (Kahn, 1974; Woodson, 1981; Zimmerman, 1972) have traced some of the origins of the phenomenon to the melting-pot character of our larger cities: Postwar emigration, for instance, has juxtaposed numerous ethnic groups in relatively narrow spaces; each group, as we are beginning to comprehend, has its own needs and methods of coping with crises. A companion factor has been the complex, variegated pattern of ways in which diverse classes and age groups are affected by the realities of modern urban life.

Another force, and a most important one, has been the loss of what Yin and Yates (1974) call "social symmetry"—the alignment of public servants and citizens and development of a sense of empathy between them. This loss of social symmetry is a principal cause of the pervasive sense of alienation that the citizen feels vis-à-vis municipal government. As Kotler, Hallman, and others have observed, the authorized or institutional linkages between the citizen and government have deteriorated to the point where the individual often feels a loss of capacity to exercise control over his or her life in the urban setting (Cunningham, 1965; Hallman, 1974; Jacobs, 1961; Kotler, 1969; Mudd, 1976). And, of course, the sense of alienation is magnified by the general problem of scale: The size of government—the total of its parts, as well as the size of its individual component agencies—very often precludes the individual's ability to identify with a government's goals and its means for reaching them.

Such concerns are at the core of the humanistic and individualistic arguments presented by Kotler and others. The gulf between the citizen and the administrative apparatus may often be ambiguous, but it is nonetheless real. Time and again, city residents complain that the government cannot be trusted, indicating quite clearly an "us and them" perspective through which perception of that chasm is expressed.

Let us face the fact that there are real inequities in the distribution of public services and resources among a city's neighborhoods. The result is a competitive climate. Alienation is further exacerbated when the residents of one neighborhood feel that they are getting less than a "fair deal" in relation to others. They articulate the problem in terms of political clout. The perception of its absence does little to enhance a neighborhood's faith in city hall or "downtown" concern or capabilities.

The impetus for decentralization is not limited to a judgment about the failure of centralized bureaucracy. There are ulterior motives at work as well, including awareness of the potential for political manipulation in decentralization efforts. Many mayors and other urban politicians have recognized the potential for political gain in decentralization programs. It is important to distinguish between pseudodecentralization drives—motivated by political self-interest—and genuine decentralization efforts; still, manipulative potential must also be understood as part of the decentralization trend.

Finally, the tendency towards decentralization has received additional impetus in the form of federal funding. The Great Society programs, with their emphasis on citizen involvement and "maximum feasible participation," established the foundation for legitimate citizen/client involvement in the program process. Besides providing a strong impetus for such participation, these requirements legitimized citizen activity and created a revolution of rising expectations among those citizens who believed they really should and could be involved in the processes by which their lives are affected.

Neighborhood decentralization is not the panacea for the delivery of mental health services. It is a realistic and feasible mechanism for addressing questions of scale. It is through the devolution of powers to neighborhood units that problems of appropriate scale can be addressed. Small is not necessarily better than large, nor is neighborhood necessarily better than city. Some functions are best organized and carried out on a regional or city level, others on a neighborhood level.

THREE APPROACHES TO NEIGHBORHOOD EMPOWERMENT

The litany of problems that is often presented to justify neighborhood empowerment and/or decentralization emerges from different ideological perspectives. Three major streams of thought have influenced the various forms of devolving power and control to neighborhoods. There are those who return to the principles of Jeffersonian democracy and the conceptual notions put forth by Lewis Mumford and Jane Jacobs to define the problem in humanistic and moral terms. They argue that centralized government increases alienation, that family and community life suffer, and that people do not cope well with the diversity and pressures of urban living (Mumford, 1968).

A second group of scholars concerned with decentralization and empowerment defines the problem within the context of American federalism, as represented by James Madison (Hallman, 1974; Ostrom, 1973; Washnis, 1972). This group builds on the theoretical framework of contemporary public administration. Their approach to the problem is functional and structural, with an emphasis on identifying the tasks that can best be carried out by small service areas (neighborhoods) and on the best means of reforming the bureaucratic infrastructure that supports current decentralization efforts. The problems are generally defined in terms of lack of accountability and limited access to services with specific concerns related to the following issues:

1. Services are unfocused and lack clear priorities.
2. Services are forced on persons unwilling to accept them.
3. Services are inaccessible to persons wanting and needing them.

4. Services are unresponsive to those needs felt most urgently by neighborhoods.
5. Service efforts are not coordinated with other social and rehabilitation programs.

Planners' preoccupation with these concerns has led to the establishment of new administrative mechanisms on the local level. These permit the public sector to exercise greater flexibility in meeting the service requirements of different types of neighborhoods. Examples of this approach include the hundreds of cities that have established neighborhood programs in crime prevention, commercial and economic revitalization, and neighborhood approaches to human and housing services. These programs are forcing city administrators to address issues of centralization and decentralization by determining which services are most effectively delivered on the neighborhood level, on the city-wide level, and on the metropolitan level. Structural and distributional issues relate to the following:

1. How resources are allocated and distributed within a city.
2. The bureaucratization of administrative and service functions.
3. The centralization of decision making and control of the city.

A third group of people concerned with the neighborhood as an arena for intellectual inquiry and service delivery are those who have their roots in the settlement house movement, the labor movement, the civil rights movement, or the Great Society programs of the 1960s. In the late nineteenth century, Jane Addams had founded Hull House, the first settlement house, in a congested section of Chicago. Here, the concern was with providing human services to the European ethnics who settled in those distressed urban neighborhoods of Chicago. As Irving Spergel has written, those who initiated the settlement house movement also developed a variety of social inventions that built upon the importance of neighborhood people in attacking social problems. "In the early 1900s the Settlement House Movement emphasized destroying the causes of dependency and degeneration through neighborhood organization" (Spergel, 1972, p. 12).

Spergel reports Elizabeth Neufeld's perception of "the establishment of social centers for the people by the people themselves. The centers were to be consumer-initiated agencies built on self-help. Miss Neufeld vigorously advocated less emphasis on institutionalism and more on decentralization and the promotion of civic neighborhood activities" (Spergel, 1972, p. 12).

In the 1930s and 1940s, activists such as Saul Alinsky pioneered in community organizing. Alinsky's roots can be traced to the stirrings of labor protest and union organizing, and the political self-assertion of the immigrants. Since then, neighborhood organizing has reached into hundreds of cities throughout the country. Tony Downs found neighborhood organizations performing the following social functions:

1. Enabling both children and adults to develop social and other skills and to increase their sense of self-worth through constructive interaction with their neighbors;
2. Providing mutual assistance concerning important aspects of daily life;
3. Pressuring government and private agencies to improve the quality and quantity of services they provide to residents of the area;
4. Providing some services to local residents that would otherwise not be furnished, or would be less suitably adapted to their needs;
5. Increasing participation of local residents in existing organizations and institutions to make them more effective in meeting the needs of those residents. (Downs, in press)

In a comprehensive analysis of community organizations in cities across the United States, Janice Perlman noted that neighborhood groups have the following approaches available to them:

1. They can use direct action to pressure existing elites and institutions for greater accountability;
2. They can seek electoral power in order to replace the existing elites and institutions;
3. They can bypass existing arrangements and establish self-help or alternative institutions such as cooperatives or community development corporations. (Perlman, 1979, p. 16)

The distinctive contribution of this philosophical orientation is that its practitioners and theorists, with roots in the social movements of this century, were concerned with the neighborhood as a locus of action for the alienated and unorganized. Discontent and alienation were two enemies that provoked action on a neighborhood basis. Whether the confrontational "militant" approach of the labor or civil rights movements was employed, or the classic enabling and developmental approach of community development practitioners was put into practice, it is clear that discontent and alienation were at issue. The neighborhood was perceived as the natural environment where problems were felt and where solutions were demanded. Consider Ross's statement in a volume on community organization theory:

Discontent with existing conditions in the community must initiate and/or nourish the development of the association; discontent must be focused and channeled into organization, planning, and action in respect to specific problems; the discontent which initiates or sustains community organization must be widely shared in the community. (Spergel, 1972, p. 14)

Regardless of which philosophical approach is dominant, it is clear that there has been a strong trend towards decentralizing services to a neighborhood level. Implicit in each ideological orientation have been issues related to control, involvement, and responsibility. The assumption is that people will live better if they have options for control; if they are involved in and take responsibility for the processes of community development.

For mental health services to become truly relevant to the needs of America's urban populace, it is necessary to identify the societal and communal processes that have led to depersonalization of human relations and intensification of the alienation process in the cities. In the next chapter a theoretical framework linking alienation and community is outlined. It is our purpose to identify the systemic origins of urban decline and the macro- and microforces responsible for conditions of alienation. We shall attempt to provide a clear conceptual framework that will assist in the operationalizing of the concepts of alienation and community in program and policy terms that the second section of this volume addresses. By relating applied and theoretical sociology to problems of orientation and empowerment, we hope to clarify vague concepts and to generate new theories and conceptual frameworks.

Greater coherence is also needed about the notion of neighborhood. It is only through an understanding of neighborhoods that we can begin to know how neighborhood networks and organizations function. By relating applied and theoretical sociology to the concept of neighborhood, we can acquire a conceptual "handle" for issues related to the empowerment process, and identify those societal and communal processes that have led to depersonalization of human relations and intensification of the alienation process in American cities.

CHAPTER 3

Alienation and Community
People, Policy, and Power

Alienation and *community* are central concepts of the modern political and social sciences. Each term is laden with value implications; each is open to a confusing array of applications. Although many studies and policy papers have employed the community or the neighborhood as their focal point, no single definition of either term has won universal acceptance. Many definitions that work well in a single theoretical construct have proven difficult in practice. The neighborhood has recently been idealized in popular culture as a bygone urban utopia, suitable for nostalgic reminiscence and panegyric, not as an arena for hard-headed political action. We have a number of useful and/or attractive definitions, none of which may be reliably employed in all circumstances. How one uses the terms obviously depends on what one wishes to do with them.

As indicated, our purpose here is to identify the processes that have led to depersonalization of human relations and intensification of the alienation process in the American urban populace, with an eye to practical remedies. We shall eventually limit our use of the concept of *community* to the context of neighborhood, employing the terms virtually interchangeably once we have clarified our understanding of them. Although our purposes require identification of the neighborhood as a geographic entity—albeit a flexibly defined entity, which can range in size from several houses on one side of a city block to a multibuilding apartment project housing a thousand people to an entire quadrant of a city in which tens of thousands of people live—we will not abandon the element of definition that declares that a community or neighborhood is also to be a shared experience. The rather poetic "we-feeling" of community may not belong exclusively to locality-based neighborhoods, but the sentiments of mutuality and common destiny that can be inferred from that element of definition deserve inclusion in any functional construct. In this instance, the public administrator, the sociologist, the social worker, and the policy maker may enhance vision through the touch of the poet.

ALIENATION: THE LONELIEST TOGETHERNESS

Much can be learned from the nineteenth century social theorists, Toennies, Marx, Weber, Durkheim, and Simmel. They provided the "context" of the twentieth century usage of the terms *alienation* and *community*. They also offer the best explanations of the authority relationship, which is central to our analysis of the potential of neighborhoods. Two strands of meaning for alienation recur throughout their writings: first, that when a person is unable to participate in, control, or understand the processes sharing his/her existence, that individual will feel deprived, dependent, and manipulated; second, that alienating conditions will arise when a community, or the institutions in that community, fail to respond to the needs of people living within that community. These two explanations will serve as our working definition of alienation.

It is our contention that the American urban populace has been experiencing feelings of powerlessness, meaninglessness, isolation, and self-estrangement; in short, a profound collective and individualized sense of alienation. In most instances, issues of devolving power to citizens on the neighborhood level in order to eliminate or decrease alienation have not been raised by social policy makers, much less dealt with. If, however, some sources of the mental health problems of much of the urban "worried well" populace can be traced to underlying neighborhood conditions that have had the effect of alienating that populace, then policies that strive to reverse or lessen the alienating elements of neighborhood life ought logically to be sought and operationalized.

A flexible enough process for defining and responding to neighborhoods' varying needs has not yet been evolved. The failure of many community mental health efforts can be traced, we believe, to the failure of the neighborhood mental health delivery system elements to confront and resolve issues involved in the devolution of power to citizens on the neighborhood level so that they, in turn, can articulate their own needs and specify practical steps towards solution of those needs.

To argue effectively for the devolution of power to people at the neighborhood level, we must first understand the functions of neighborhoods in urban life. Alienation, we recognize, is the condition in need of remedy. The neighborhood, we contend, is the context in which that remedy ought to be applied.

THE TOENNIES TYPOLOGIES

It was Ferdinand Toennies who provided the conceptual typology that made it possible to clearly distinguish between the *communal* and *noncommunal* process. Toennies not only provided a classification analysis, but through his differentiation of *gemeinschaft* and *gesellschaft* as types of social organization, he provided a sociological explanation of alienation in the context of capitalism, and the modern bureaucratic state. Toennies's seminal classificatory structure provided a basis on which Weber, Durkheim, Marx, Simmel, and other students of community could build theoretical explanations, thus providing greater understanding of the massive social changes affecting community life and society (Toennies, 1887/1957).

It should be observed that the *gemeinschaft* and the *gesellschaft* represent idealized types, not actual descriptions of actual communities. *Gemeinschaft* easily translates into "community" or even "neighborhood." The family is the basis of life in the *gemeinschaft*. Village and town are regarded as extended families containing a variety of formal and informal helping networks and support systems. The reliance of people upon one another arises spontaneously from the particular identity and/or situation they share.

By contrast, the city is typified by the *gesellschaft*. Commerce is the dominant factor here. Capital wealth, or money, is the only important resource. The only characteristic effectively differentiating people from one another is their wealth. The extent of one's freedom correlates with the extent of one's wealth. Helping networks and support systems are irrelevant. Associations are forged by self-interest, by rational calculations of gains and losses, and by impersonal criteria of merit. Whereas the cohesion of the *gemeinschaft* is rooted in diffuse sympathy, the people of the *gesellschaft* are melded into a unit by bureaucratic rules and formal mechanisms of social control.

Each of the nineteenth century scholars cited earlier has regarded the bureaucratic state as the principal source of human alienation. A scholarly debate over communal and noncommunal explanations of human alienation continues to this day. There is, however, general agreement on the factors that have contributed to the breakdown of urban neighborhoods in America. These include industrialization,

rapid urbanization, fluctuating patterns of migration, and macroeco-
nomic forces. Not so familiar, however, are various proposals for solutions to these issues.

IN SEARCH OF A SENSE OF NEIGHBORHOOD[1]

As we have stated repeatedly, community mental health planners
have never developed their services within the context of a real sense
of neighborhood. This is understandable. Urban neighborhoods are
complex entities. Few planners and policy analysts have been trained
to understand them and their workings. But, what is a neighborhood?
The question of how we define a neighborhood is not easily answered
nor agreed upon by researchers and scholars.
    Roland Warren has observed that:

> Life would be much simpler for students of the subject if communities could
> be clearly delineated geographically from each other, and if there was no
> overlapping among them. But this is not the case. The community concept,
> based as it is on common life shared by people within a specific geographic
> area, presents both practical and theoretical difficulties once one attempts
> to draw lines on a map. It is relatively easy to define and delimit an orga-
> nization, or a business company, or a governmental unit. The community
> remains elusive, often encompassing one area and one group of people if
> looked at in a certain way, a different area and different people if looked at
> in another. (R. Warren, 1963, p. 8)

NEIGHBORHOOD AS TERRITORY

Neighborhoods traditionally have been thought of either in terms
of physical characteristics or social relationships. Ruth Glass in 1948
defined neighborhood from a planning perspective as a distinctive territorial group, distinct by virtue of the specific physical characteristics
of the area and the specific social characteristics of the inhabitants
(Hojnacki, 1979).
    The territorial or geographical aspect of neighborhood was empha-
sized as early as 1915 in the work of Robert Park. Park viewed a city in
terms of concentric zones emerging around central downtown. He
argued that each zone, or neighborhood, has a specific characteristic
that distinguishes it from other subareas within a city. The work of
scholars following Park's tradition kept area as a basic unit of analysis,

---

[1]This section is principally based on D. Biegel, *Help-Seeking and Receiving in Urban
Ethnic Neighborhoods.* Unpublished doctoral dissertation, University of Maryland,
1982.

but brought in more social flavor. Shevsky and Bell (1950) used their "social area analysis" technique to examine social, economic, and cultural aspects of urban neighborhoods.

There is little consensus thought on what constitutes physical boundaries for a given neighborhood. Peter Mann (1970), in his essay "The Neighborhood," wrote, "A person has neighbors and, therefore, the limits of his acquaintance may be said to limit his neighborhood." This implies that neighborhoods have no fixed boundaries. Several empirical studies support this assertion. For example, Roos and Broden (1976), in a study based on interviews with 200 residents, found 50 different boundaries of a neighborhood. While they found little agreement concerning the boundaries of the neighborhood, they did find that two-thirds of their sample responded by giving a specific neighborhood name, and thus, had a definite perception of living in an identifiable neighborhood. Morris and Hess (1975) view the boundaries of a neighborhood as that which is easily walked by the residents so that going from one side to another does not require special effort. Other research indicates that many residents, especially the elderly, view their neighborhood as only one block (Biegel & Sherman, 1979).

Hojnacki (1979) reports on a study by Richard Coleman of the Joint Center for Urban Studies of MIT and Harvard. Coleman feels that there are hierarchical levels of neighborhood identification. He found that there are different graduations in the geographic definition of neighborhood, each with a different social and symbolic meaning. The first level of identification is a small circle surrounding one's home. The second level of identification often overlaps with recognizable neighborhood names and sociocultural homogeneity. The final level is one of the identification with large and diverse geographical names.

Neighborhoods as Social and Political Entities

The social interaction aspect of neighborhoods is emphasized in the work of Caplow and Forman (1950), Litwak and Szelenyi (1969), and others. Caplow and Forman defined neighborhood as: A family dwelling unit and the ten family dwelling units most accessible to it. Physical proximity thus limits social relationships. Similarly, Litwak and Szelenyi contend that neighborhoods derive their unique functions and characteristics from face-to-face contact and interaction among neighbors. They identify three functions of this interaction with neighbors. The first is the opportunity for quick or immediate involvement. The extent of such interactions may be as simple as borrowing a cup of sugar in the middle of preparing a meal, or as complex as rescuing a neighbor from an unforeseen disaster. The second function is related to receiving and improving services through organizational participation. For example, people living in the same area have common needs and problems pertaining to sanitation, police protection, education, and so forth. Cooperative interaction with neighbors can help to improve these services. The third function of face-to-face contact is socialization. Neighborly contact gives rise to internalized learning of such norms as how to be a good mother, how to dress, definition of delinquent behavior, and so on. Organizational participation and the socialization process serve, in fact, to encourage the integration of individuals in the community (Caplow & Forman, 1950; Keller, 1968; Litwak, 1961).

Susan Keller, in reviewing previous literature, found a general agreement that neighborhoods consist of both geographic and social components. Other than these two characteristics, however, neighborhood attributes are not clearly defined. She defined neighborhood in terms of four elements. According to Keller:

> Essentially it [neighborhood] refers to distinctive areas into which larger spatial units may be subdivided—the distinctiveness of these areas stems from different sources whose independent contributions are difficult to assess: geographical boundaries, ethnic or cultural characteristics of the inhabitants, psychological unity among people who feel that they belong together, or concentrated use of an area's facilities for shopping, leisure, and learning. (Keller, 1968, p. 87)

The concentrated and distinctive use that Keller notes of shops, schools, and parks by neighborhood residents may serve indirectly to link neighbors to one another and to the area, giving rise to neighborhood attachments. Such attachments serve important psychosocial functions for individual well-being (Bowlby, 1977). As Warren notes, the concept of neighborhood and attachment becomes a crucial element in the study of social interaction.

> When all such difficulties are considered, a few sociologists throw up their hands and urge that the whole concept of the community be discarded as a sort of useless theoretical will-o'-the-wisp. Yet the term remains, and community analysis goes forward. The reason is simple. People's lives and their behavior are significantly influenced by their propinquity. Living together in close physical proximity calls for social structures and social functions which sustain life in the locality and provide the satisfactions which people seek. By living in the same geographical area, even in today's conditions of rapid transportation, people must share common local institutions and facilities. They have a common interest in the local schools, stores, sources of employment, churches, and other institutions and services whose availability to individuals in their own locality is a part of the total pattern of American society. The intertwining of their lives on a locality basis, even in these days of specialized interests, urban anonymity, and depersonalization, pro-

vides an important social reality and an important focus of study, fraught with theoretical difficulty though such study may be. We shall see in the following chapter that several new approaches to community study, as well as the best in some of the older approaches, provide tools for a meaningful analysis of such locality-oriented behavior. (R. Warren, 1963, p. 9)

For Morris and Hess (1975), neighborhood is really a dual concept: (1) an image in the minds of those living there or the way outsiders view the area; and (2) the resources and physical dimensions that character-ize it.

Classifying Neighborhood Types

Although distinct territorial, sociocultural and psychological dimensions are evident, the concept of neighborhood may be more complex than that. Roland Warren (1977), in his *New Perspectives on the American Community,* states that neighborhoods or local commu-nities are distinguishable along a complex set of dimensions, including primary group relations, autonomy, viability, distribution of power, degree of participation, commitment, degree of heterogeneity, extent of neighborhood control, and extent of conflict (p. 2).

Donald Warren (1977; Warren & Clifford, 1975), based on NIMH-funded field research in the Detroit metropolitan area, developed a typology of neighborhoods focused around helping networks. He iden-tified six types of neighborhoods on the basis of their social organiza-tions and reference orientations:

1. *Integrated.* People in this neighborhood are very cohesive. Neighbors know and interact with each other, and people belong to many organizations within and without the neighborhood.
2. *Parochial.* There is an extensive amount of contact with neigh-bors that is face-to-face, but also an absence of ties to the larger community. This type of neighborhood is protective of its status and tries to enforce conformity to its own cultural system.
3. *Diffuse.* Informal and face-to-face social participation is lack-ing. The structure of this neighborhood may produce intra-neighborhood conflict.
4. *Stepping Stone.* This type of neighborhood has social institu-tions to integrate the newcomer quickly. However, conflict may arise between the goals of the neighborhood and the values of socially mobile residents.
5. *Transitory.* Residents do not participate in or identify with a local community. There is a lack of neighborhood structure and

people generally keep to themselves. Residents are concerned
with the mobility of their families.
6. *Anomie Neighborhood.* This neighborhood is disorganized and
lacks participation patterns and a sense of identification with
local or large community.

The major views on the nature of neighborhoods cited thus far
have been sociological. An alternative way of viewing neighborhood
functions is in terms of social change, governance, and public policy.
Morris and Hess (1975), for example, view neighborhoods as building
blocks of democracy. Naparstek (1976), with reference to the work of
Jacobs (1961), Cunningham (1965), and Morris and Hess (1975), states
his thesis that failure to include neighborhoods as a partner in public
policy decisions increases alienation and has negative impact on family
and community life. Others (Ahlbrandt & Cunningham, 1979; Cutright,
1977; Dennis & Geruson, 1977; Martineau, 1977) have agreed that each
neighborhood is a unique entity—unique in resident commitment, satisfaction, social fabric, availability of neighborhood-based institutions,
racial, ethnic, economic, and other characteristics—and that neighborhoods must be utilized as a force in public policy. Given such diversity,
policy made exclusively in Washington, D.C., is bound to fail.

Paul Levy (1979), in an attempt to integrate previous research on
neighborhoods, has identified three roles of neighborhoods: (1) neighborhood as a power base; (2) neighborhood as a social base; and (3)
neighborhood as a political base. Without question, we have seen since
the 1960s a tremendous growth in neighborhood consciousness and
power through the development on the local level of thousands of
neighborhood-based advocacy organizations and self-help groups.

Some scholars (Berger & Neuhaus, 1977; Greer, 1968) have concluded that neighborhoods defy definition. Berger and Neuhaus state
flatly that a neighborhood is in fact what the people who are there say
it is. Whatever frame of reference for the concept of neighborhood
eventually emerges, it must certainly be a flexible one. The literature
suggests that the major orientations towards neighborhood include: the
territorial or geographic orientation—regarding the community as a
spatial entity; the humanistic orientation—regarding the community as
a localized population sharing certain institutions and values; the functional orientation—analyzing the community via the associations or
interactions of local people with one another and their behavior in
regard to one another; the economic orientation—consideration of the
community in terms of its power structure; and the sociocultural
conceptualization.

Roland Warren's analysis, however, melds the major attitudes about neighborhoods, builds on Toennies's ideal types, and provides theoretical underpinnings for defining neighborhood helping networks, and linking the neighborhood to the outside world. In his analysis of community functions, Warren differentiates the vertical and horizontal patterns of relationships in which single elements within localized communities are involved. The vertical pattern accounts for the structural and functional relationships of local social units with each other. Both patterns of functioning are viewed as essential though frequently incomplete. There is a rough correspondence between the vertical pattern and task function—getting things done—and between the horizontal pattern and system maintenance (R. Warren, 1963).

Warren observes that the values, goals, and norms of behavior of the vertical and horizontal patterns tend not to coincide, although individuals within a single community may find themselves involved in simultaneous relationships with both conflicting systems. Vital extracommunity ties can be found within a community's diverse component units, which are themselves units of an extracommunity system. In circumstances where the demands of the two systems are incompatible, Warren has found that the vertical ties are generally stronger. There is a mutual tendency for vertical ties to strengthen and for new vertical ties to develop between a local unit and extracommunity systems. The tendency accounts for what Warren terms "The Great Change": "the orientation of local units or extra-community systems in American society."

Warren describes two models for the flow of authority in the vertical pattern; down from the geographically larger and functionally more inclusive unit, or up from relatively autonomous units that form a relatively loose confederation. His discussion of a community's horizontal pattern, he says, is "what holds the whole thing together on the local level." While the vertical pattern corresponds roughly to Toennies's gesellschaft, the horizontal pattern is similarly related to Toennies's gemeinschaft. The network of horizontal associations within a neighborhood provides the cement that "holds the whole thing together." The individual associations within the horizontal pattern serve as mediating structures to the rest of society.

NECESSARY LINKS: THE NEIGHBORHOOD AND EXTRACOMMUNITY SYSTEMS

Yet the solution to America's urban crisis is not to be found exclusively at the level of the local neighborhood associations. The functioning of the gemeinschaft is essential to the well-being of neighborhood residents, but the operation of the *gesellschaft* impacts importantly on them as well. It would be naive to overlook or underestimate these forces in neighborhood life. One of the most comprehensive studies of the impact of economic forces and governmental policies on local communities may be found in a soon-to-be-published study by Anthony Downs entitled *Understanding Neighborhoods* (in press). Downs traces the effects of federal, state, and city policies on neighborhoods. He analyzes how economic growth and stagnation in the macrosociety affect the internal structure of neighborhood communities. An extracommunity decision—made, say, by an automobile manufacturer in Detroit—can impact upon the internal structure and the well-being of a neighborhood and its people in an entirely different city. Most importantly, Downs demonstrates that the same enormous diversity of urban conditions in the United States precludes the possibility of one single set of policies effectively coping with the problems of every metropolitan area, city, or neighborhood. Key choices, then, in determining the policies for each place need to be made at the metropolitan—area, city, and neighborhood—levels, not at the national and state levels. How such metropolitan decision-making can take place without being undermined by the civil service administrator class remains an unsolved political problem. Perhaps awareness at the appropriate level of solution and the nature of the problem will forewarn elected officials and other key decision makers.

PARTNERSHIPS FOR MENTAL HEALTH

It is our contention that the neighborhood context represents the most appropriate and promising level for the design and operation of community mental health programs for the "worried well" and the sick who need social support while they are in remission. The neighborhood/community context holds particular promise for the treatment of persons whose mental health conditions have arisen as a result of the widespread alienation in America's urban centers. The placement of the power and responsibility for development and supervision of community mental health services—particularly those for the "worried well," who do not require high-technology psychiatric care—in the hands of locally empowered neighborhood groups will have the further effect of strengthening them, increasing their capacity for self-help, and reducing their sense of alienation from the larger society.

Yet this devolution of power to neighborhood groups cannot be successful if only a modicum of resources and a full measure of responsibilities are simply "dumped" on them. In isolation, community groups and networks have neither the funding nor the expertise to do the whole job. Neighborhood people are best qualified to define their specific needs and to design programs that will work best for them in meeting those needs. But the relationships of the units within a single neighborhood to extracommunity systems are also essential to the operation of local units within that community. Our systems operate independently when they operate effectively. Functional partnerships must be formulated between local groups involved in community mental health, and the city, state, and national mental health systems, as well as the professionals involved in the care of the mentally ill and the prevention of mental illness.

This book is based on a process method from which we have drawn examples and policy implications of neighborhood empowerment. The empowerment model itself is contained in chapter 7. In chapter 4 we shall review some relevant mental health and human service policy developments of the recent past.

We contend that the community health movement has not provided services for either the "worried well" or the severely ill on a *human scale.* The theme and substance of this volume is that human scale services demand the use of human scale institutions. One key must be the neighborhoods in which humans reside, work, play, and create mutual support structures. Community support system programs cannot be dropped into neighborhoods from high-flying federal cargo planes. Community institutions must be fostered to grow naturally within their neighborhood setting. Most important, the professional and the planner must avoid the mistake of seeing neighborhood empowerment and high technology hospitals as being necessarily in conflict. There is nothing particularly humane about leaving a human being to suffer in a lonely boarding house when the technology to mitigate his misery could be available in a regional hospital. Bridging the gap between the neighborhood and the mental health facility is crucial both to early case finding and to postdischarge rehabilitation. In the models presented in this book, many individuals will be seen to receive support within their neighborhoods and without ever having to be labeled as "patients." For the 3% who require the services of a mental health care system, the key is excellence in human technological intervention and linkages to crucial neighborhood resources.

Most of us will someday find that our homes have at least temporarily become places of tension and need. Meaningful neighborhood structures can and ought to be empowered to help us. The loneliness and alienation of this age of anxiety must in time give way to a new era of communal support systems and helping networks that operate on a genuinely human scale, in partnership with professional systems for care delivery.

How we got to where we are is the preoccupation of the following chapter, a critical overview of the progress—and lack of progress—that has resulted from federal attempts to guide or provide mental health service, and parallel attempts to establish a system of human services to serve the neediest segments of American society.

CHAPTER 4

Cycles and Circles

An Overview of Federal Policies in Mental Health and Human Services

Few themes in health and social policy are really new; certainly interest in the relationship between care of the mentally ill and the community is neither new nor an exclusively Western preoccupation.[1] This chapter presents a brief review of the development of policies concerned with mental health and human services in the United States, and raises questions about the future.

GOING THE FULL CIRCLE: FROM "THE COMMUNITY IS THE PROBLEM" TO "THE COMMUNITY IS THE SOLUTION"

In the early nineteenth century, mental health care in the United States was focused on the insane. The insane were removed from the chaotic conditions of Jacksonian society, which were felt to be partially to blame for their insanity, and placed in the controlled, ordered, and secure environment of the asylum located far from the community. Asylums attempted to create islands of refuge and humane care. The treatment philosophy was known as "moral treatment." The tremendous growth of asylums during this period was enhanced by the campaigns of such reformers as Dorthea Dix against iniquitous and cruel abuse of the mentally ill. No one who has read Dix's work or the work of other pre-Civil War reformers can romanticize "neighborhood care"

[1]Initial findings of the World Survey of Schizophrenia suggest that the lower prevalence of the disorder in non-Western cultures may be traceable to superior family and community support systems. The Chinese approach to mental health emphasizes the same factors. Before its 1979 revolution, Iran reported very similar mental health problems in its cities as those identified in American cities.

31

or remain unaware of the dangers of dumping desperately ill human beings into communities with neither adequate support systems nor bridges to proper medical and psychiatric facilities. Contrary to popular mythology, the state hospital did not replace warm, loving family care in an intimate neighborhood structure. Care was separated early from the neighborhood and the family, and delegated to almshouses and poor farms into which were herded together the young and old, epileptic, feeble-minded, and insane. (Over 150 of the asylums created between 1810 and 1860 remain in place to this day.)

The growth of cities in the United States after the Civil War was fed by waves of immigration. Extended family support systems and traditional multigeneration neighborhood structures that may enhance care of the mentally ill in rural communities were not dominant in the new ethnic neighborhoods. Despite improvements in hospital planning during the Kirkbride era, problems mounted.

It is not within the scope of this chapter to review the decay and failure of moral therapy and the snakepits that subsequently emerged in thoroughly planned state hospitals. Their fate may be briefly summarized: too many patients, too little money, too few staff, alienation from community ties, class and ethnic prejudices, and disintegration of treatment programming. The original model was based on the notion that the community may cause illness and the asylum may cure illness. Paradoxically, the latest battle cry has been that asylums may cause illness and communities may cure illness. For the severely ill, problems of too many patients, too little money, too few staff, and alienation from neighborhoods recur with both models.

By the turn of the twentieth century, a movement developed that viewed the community as both a source of the problem and a component of the potential solution. Seeds of the community mental health movement were being planted. Dr. Adolph Meyer of the Johns Hopkins University Hospital, who did pioneering work in community mental health at the beginning of the century, believed that effective treatment of mental health problems would require a focus on environmental and community factors.

The mental hygiene movement was a significant effort to bring to bear newly developing theories of human behavior at a community level. Orthopsychiatry was particularly related to prevention of emotional disorders through improvement of parenting and early treatment of emotional disorders in children. The movement floundered once more on the realities of long waiting lists, promises that exceeded available technology, and underfunding. The creation of what Leon Eisenbert has described as the new "Holy Trinity"—the psychiatrist, the psychologist, and the social worker—meant that the time-consuming, extensive "multidisciplinary" evaluation was often succeeded by labeling and a deficient treatment system. Whereas some psychiatric social workers were successful in linking with neighborhood schools, recreation workers, churches, and clubs, too often the community was ignored.

World War II brought a new wave of concern about mental illness. More than 10% of draftees were found to be suffering from major psychiatric disorders. A generation of young physicians working under General William Menninger found new ways to intervene effectively in traumatic neuroses. Post-World War II studies established the importance of group morale and effective leadership in the occurrence of combat neuroses. In the post-World War II era, the National Institute of Mental Health (NIMH) was created. A major research and education effort was launched. In less than a decade and a half, the psychiatric manpower pool was increased fourfold. Clinical psychology, psychiatric social work, and psychiatric nursing also flourished during this period.

THE EMERGING FEDERAL ROLE IN MENTAL HEALTH

The 1950s saw a revival of community concerns as this new wave of professionals sought to grapple with the problems of mental illness. A halfway house movement began in the mid-1950s even before the phenothiazine revolution. In the late 1950s, a national commission produced a landmark volume, *Action for Mental Health*, which emphasized the importance of community ties to enable patients to reenter community structures (Joint Commission on Mental Illness & Health, 1961). *Action for Mental Health* gave impetus to the modern community mental health movement, which was officially born with the passage of the Community Mental Health Centers (CMHC) Act in 1963. Before this law, responsibility for mental health care was primarily placed with the states. Most of the mentally ill were cared for in understaffed and underfunded state hospitals, hospitals which provided more custody than treatment. Introducing his bill in a speech to Congress in 1963, President John F. Kennedy stated that it was to be "a bold, new approach." The CMHC Act seemed far-reaching and revolutionary. The treatment locus would shift from the state hospital to sites closer to the community. "This approach," Kennedy stated, "relies primarily upon the new knowledge and the new drugs acquired and developed in recent years which make it possible for most of the mentally ill to be successfully and quickly treated in their communities and returned to a useful place in society." The new legislation was widely acclaimed and praised in professional and community circles. Mental health care had come full circle in a century and a half, from a negative view of "community" to a positive view, and from "institutional" to "community-based" care and treatment.

The 1963 Kennedy legislation, which funded only construction of mental health centers, and the subsequent staffing laws represented a federal initiative to bring treatment of acute illness close enough to community structures to facilitate secondary and tertiary prevention. Much pseudohistory has been written reconstructing what was actually intended. Remote, massive, overcrowded state institutions were to be succeeded by an integrated system of care. Accessibility and continuity were the watchwords. The presence of outpatient, inpatient, day hospital, emergency, and consultation and education programs were to provide comprehensive treatment.

Neither the 1960s legislation nor *Action for Mental Health* promised to stamp out mental illness through primary prevention. Neither the strategy nor the technology of primary prevention has evolved sufficiently to support such a promise. The leaders of the 1950s and the 1960s knew this. Their successors in the 1980s are no less cautious with their promises. Anyone who reads *Action for Mental Health* as a promise that neighborhood empowerment will stamp out schizophrenia and depressive illness is seriously misreading what is written there. Elsewhere we have described in detail the issues and opportunities that surround direct prevention issues (Spiro, 1980b).

The promise of the 1960s was establishment of neighborhood linkages to enhance care. That promise has remained, by and large, unmet.

Perhaps the main failure was in the conceptualization of the emotional disturbances. This often drifted into wishful thinking and naive formulation. Mint-fresh graduates of mental health professional schools were often set loose on severely ill schizophrenics with no better formulation than "labeling makes them crazy." Illnesses with established genetic transmission patterns were viewed as mere reactions to stresses of everyday life. Many centers were equipped only to deal with the "worried well." Under the banner of deinstitutionalization, the seriously ill were dumped out of grim state hospitals in sylvan settings into grim boarding homes and nursing homes in city slums. It was a movement out of the snakepit and into the gutter. Communication between state hospitals and local communities was often very poor. Community services were never designed and, as a result, were ill prepared to deal with patients with the level of illness of those being discharged from state hospitals. The whole issue of severe, chronic mental illness was treated as though it were simply a product of institutionalization. Thus, individuals who suffered from Gruenberg's chronic social breakdown syndrome were confused with severe psychotics whose natural illness would remain severe no matter where they were kept. There were elements of cynicism, even destructiveness, in the deinstitutionalization movement (Spiro, 1982).

CURRENT POLICY CONCERNS

The "bold, new approach" of the 1960s has become the target of significant attacks by both consumers and professionals. Among the criticisms leveled against the community mental health movement have been the following issues: lack of coordination of services; fragmentation of services; lack of accessibility of services; lack of utilization of services; problems of accountability; barriers to care; professionals' lack of understanding of community; insufficient manpower; and problems of evaluation (Agranoff, 1977; Bindman, 1966; Caplan & Grunebaum, 1967; Gordon, 1977; Klein, 1969; Naparstek & Biegel, 1982; President's Commission on Mental Health, 1978; Rieff, 1966; Schiff, 1973). At the end of the revolutionary series of changes in the 1960s, Spiro argued that for all the problems of the community mental health centers, they still represented a significant improvement over the state hospital systems they were intended to replace. He urged that community mental health centers should be judged against this standard rather than just some El Dorado fantasy system that no person has yet conceived or implemented (Spiro, 1969). Still, even such proponents of community mental health centers as Spiro urged that the community mental health center move out in new directions: towards tertiary care institutions that give high-technology and highly specialized care when it is indicated, and towards true neighborhood structures through neighborhood programs.

In retrospect, it would appear that the lack of linkages to neighborhood networks and support systems has been a central stumbling block. The term *community* in community mental health has been a misnomer from the beginning. The service or *catchment* area for the community mental health system of the 1960s and 1970s has been a sometimes capriciously and arbitrarily designated aggregate of between 75,000 and 200,000 persons. There has been little or no conceptualization of real neighborhoods in the original proposals, and little more recognition of neighborhood has emerged since. In fact, mental health catchment areas have sometimes split neighborhoods in half, weakening rather than strengthening or building on existing support systems.

The present reality of the public sector's role in the delivery of mental health services has produced the conviction that "things are not working." A case in point is the deinstitutionalization mess, an attempt to link the state hospital system to the community mental health system. Hundreds of thousands of former mental patients have been released from hospitals across the nation since 1963 under a federal reform policy that alleged that institutions did as much harm as good. Federal mental health planners envisioned the flowering of a network of supportive care for the deinstitutionalized patients at the community level through the stimulus of federal seed money. But 1,200 of the 2,000 community mental health centers projected for 1980 failed to materialize, and many that were created failed to service this chronically ill target population. Planners, without consultation, assumed that strong neighborhoods could accept the chronically ill. When few welcomed large numbers of these troubled people, patients were steered to transitional neighborhoods that would not put up a fuss. Here the strong community support factor essential for successful aftercare was absent. City streets became the wards of mental hospitals (Naparstek & Biegel, 1979; Spiro, 1982).

In the 1970s, as it became increasingly apparent that human scale services were not emerging, other federal initiatives received emphasis. One approach was to increase the number of mandated services from five to twelve. Aftercare, service to children, service to alcoholics and the chemically dependent, services to the elderly, rehabilitation, and so forth, were mandated. The net effect was to burden community mental health centers with obligations that could not possibly be met at the neighborhood level.

THE IDEA OF A COMPREHENSIVE SYSTEM OF CARE

Slowly, in the late 1970s, federal planners began to realize that only through the evolution of a truly comprehensive mental health care system could all of these various services be provided. Even in the 1960s, proposals had been made for a tri-level care system (Spiro, 1969). The tri-level care system proposed in this theoretical paper was elaborated in the City of Milwaukee between 1975 and 1980. By utilizing this method, it was possible, quietly, to focus neighborhood services through true neighborhood structures. Unfortunately, in other cities, evolving community mental health centers spent more time, resources, energy, and money in proliferating thinly manned services than they did on empowering neighborhoods to provide self-help programs. Burgeoning inspection and paperwork further contributed to the creation of top-heavy bureaucratic institutions. Accountability, the catchword of the 1970s, came to mean reams of paperwork and minimal measurement of actual function. Slowly, the community mental health center drifted out of the care of clinicians and community experts and into the hands of a new managerial class. These same trends may obliterate progress in Milwaukee even as this volume is being written.

Increasing problems of fragmentation gave rise to "case manager" approaches in an effort to help patients and clients negotiate their way through complex mental health resources and neighborhood human service and health resources. As more and more individual professionals were responsible for the client, the client was more and more likely to fall between the cracks. As the old adage goes, "When everyone is responsible, in effect, no one is responsible."

Federal policy in general health care delivery has paralleled mental health policy with even more negative effects. Hill–Burton Legislation produced many investments in secondary care suburban hospital beds and the abandonment of many central-city resources. Policies for primary and tertiary care resources have failed to develop from the original legislation. The layering of care was actually disrupted. Outmoded, center-city hospital emergency rooms became the loci of primary care for many neighborhoods. The flight of doctors from core cities was actually encouraged by poorly designed government health aid to the indigent. The mass media heightened the disincentives to remain downtown by publishing lists of names of physicians receiving Title XIX and Title XVIII payments.

A patchwork crazy quilt of badly planned "control" mechanisms was rushed into place to hold costs down. The control mechanisms have been ineffective in cost control, have removed free-market effectiveness—which could close some hospitals—and are in themselves very costly. No noticeable reform has been produced to date.

These poorly conceived policies have had a marked effect on mental health care. They slowed natural tendencies to rid society of costly, inefficient, government-run hospitals that the private sector could have—and should have—replaced. Physical plant and equipment have degenerated so badly, thanks to the inappropriate red tape of Health Systems Agencies (HSAs), that inpatient costs have risen much higher than they need to be. Because Title XIX pays for the mentally ill in general hospitals, but not in specialty private psychiatric hospitals, high-technology care has slipped away from the promising therapeutic communities of the 1960s to pure disease-control and high-cost facilities. HSAs have produced chaos in mental health care through enforcement of rules irrelevant to mental health care by persons untainted by knowledge or training in mental health.

But the most serious effect has been the creation of yet another new form of snakepit—total institution; the skilled nursing facilities (SNFs) nursing home. As programs follow the health dollars, potential Title XIX patients have been moved out of facilities with reasonable recreation and therapeutic community model resources to buildings constructed and staffed according to largely inappropriate physical-disease, nursing-home codes. The elderly, the physically handicapped, and young schizophrenics have at times been indiscriminately mixed in entrepreneurial profit-making nursing homes devoid of a trained mental health staff. Nursing homes have been created in a pattern disregarding transitional communities and have often developed with the worst features of total institutions. Physical and chemical restraints have replaced the concept of safe haven. This hodge-podge incurred by bad federal health policies has passed for "community care" and "deinstitutionalization."

Insurance payment patterns, hospital construction regulations, and health cost control mechanisms markedly affect patterns of mental health care. Despite escalating costs disproportionate with inflation, services are growing worse, not better. The heavy hand of government and bureaucratic regulation is found wherever one turns. Money is wasted on the "regulators" that should go towards neighborhood empowerment and high-technology care by experts.

DISTINGUISHING SOCIAL MALADJUSTMENT FROM MENTAL ILLNESS

Mental health care was assumed to be a subset of "human services" in the 1960s and 1970s, thanks to poorly documented speculation that *all* major mental illness is the product of social pressures, poverty, social roles, or untoward labeling.

Lumping severe illnesses with social maladjustments that could be dealt with in neighborhood structures has had the effect of producing a sense of despair and nihilism unjustified by available evidence. The "worried well," who have sustained social maladjustment, may certainly be aided effectively through neighborhood structures, but the severely ill require both high-technology care and subsequent social support.

Federal policy has been ineffectual on two levels. It has failed to take into account the special needs of persons with major psychiatric illnesses and may even have increased the stigma attached to such persons when they are dumped, uncared for, into their neighborhoods. Simultaneously, federal policy has failed to realize the potential of neighborhoods in producing support structures and aid for problems of daily living. This has had the dual effect of separating the "worried well" from their neighborhoods and institutionalizing their care in inappropriate settings. Simultaneously, the severely ill patients were relabeled "clients," were offered inappropriate support nostrums, discarded into rooming houses, and removed from real sources of needed high-technology psychiatric care.

The problems of the community mental health movement are not unique to mental health, but are characteristic of the entire human services delivery system. Let us now consider some major social policy trends in human service during this century in America.

OVERVIEW: HUMAN SERVICES

In the early 1900s, human services were provided by such neighborhood-based organizations as the settlement houses and the political ward clubs. As society became more complex, well intentioned reforms were carried out by professionals in government. The result was the establishment of secular institutions to help individuals to function more adequately. Although the public sector dominance in human service and mental health service delivery was a major and positive breakthrough in terms of government's responsibility to those in need, the change created many problems. The traditional ties to the neighborhood had been broken, and large, impersonal, bureaucratic institutions increasingly dominated the human service domain.

In order to effect change, we need to understand how and why current service patterns occurred. Federal involvement in the human services began in the early years of the twentieth century when progressive and labor movement leadership focused public attention on the impact that the industrial revolution had on children and families. Federal initiatives soon followed as labor and political leaders urged the federal government to establish the Children's Bureau, vocational education programs, and maternal and child health programs. Each federal service initiative was linked to state government, but the principal providers of organized human services were still the wide array of private charitable organizations.

The Great Depression of the 1930s forced the national government to redefine its role; and with the passage of the Social Security Act, the federal government had the statutory framework for providing direct income support payments and, subsequently, direct services to designated groups of people, such as the elderly, the disabled, the blind, and dependent children.

Francis Perkins, as noted by Theodore Lowi, believed that Social Security was framed in a context of fear:

> Fear had made a welfare program of some sort necessary; fear had also made it politically possible.... We would not have had Social Security without the crisis of the depression. (Lowi, 1969, p. 218)

Lowi states that, through the crisis of the Depression and the fear of insurrection, the nation fundamentally changed its ideology and moved away from a purely residual conception of welfare, challenging the puritanical concept of poverty. Poverty was no longer perceived merely as a result of individual sin, sloth, and incompetence. Now economic and social factors were accepted as contributing causes. In this fashion, the Social Security Act of 1935 initiated a national effort to provide income maintenance and services to a large segment of the nation's population.

Sundquist indicates that the legislation of the New Deal separated poor people into two categories: the able-bodied unemployed, for whom jobs were the solution, and those who were unable to work, for whom financial assistance was provided. He states:

> This dichotomy led to the acceptance of two great national objectives. One of these was full employment for all who were able and seeking work.... The other was a minimum decent standard of living, through Social Security, for those in need and not able to work—the children of fatherless households, the old, the disabled. (Sundquist, 1968, p. 112)

Thus, the precarious ideological balance would be resolved through the national workings of the economy and, if so needed, residual programs for those who could not participate in the marketplace. Prior to the 1960s, the social problems associated with poverty would be attacked directly but through overly specific, piecemeal programs— urban renewal would clear the slums, youth work would cope with juvenile delinquency, public housing would improve the shelter of the poor, and so on (Sundquist, 1968).

Critics of human services during the later 1940s, and through the 1950s, were preoccupied with the overuse of services by small numbers of "multiproblem families." Rein's thoughtful summary of casework practice during this time provides some useful insight:

> At one time, it was felt that the caseworkers relied on a narrow conception that emphasized client readiness and willingness to use the formally scheduled office interviews. This had the effect of excluding low income families who could not conform to these standards. In response to this criticism, aggressive casework developed in the 1950's, where workers were encouraged to reach out into the community in search of their clients. But the results of these efforts were not altogether beneficient; for as Alvin Schorr observed, it leads to intrusion, direction, and coercion in the lives of clients. (Rein, 1970, p. 113)

Rein further points to a series of studies that extended the criticism of the human services as practiced prior to the early 1960s. Critical issues raised by the research were: the labeling and rejection of the poor by social service agencies; the tendency of agencies to work with "good" clients, as opposed to those who were the poorest, the least motivated, or perhaps the sickest; the discriminatory use of staff in terms of the least competent staff working with clients who were the most socially incompetent. In addition, the social services were found incapable of helping clients to utilize community institutions that would help them find better jobs. And perhaps the most devastating finding directed at the human services was that "they were not only rigid and indifferent to the needs of their clients but actually *harmful* to them. A cultural gulf between the professional and the consumer had developed" (Rein, 1970, p. 335).

A laissez-faire orientation toward dealing with poverty seems to have been a basic premise of the Eisenhower administration. Marris and Rein note that the administration had faith that the institutional aspects of the economy would resolve the problems associated with poverty. They state:

> The early years of President Eisenhower's conservative administration had been sustained by the doctrine that economic growth would itself, by diffusing prosperity, reduce inequalities and resolve social problems. The standard of living for all seemed to be rising, and the position of the unskilled improved more rapidly than others. The progressive tax structure, expanded welfare services, mass public education, and the G.I. Bill all served the twin aims of economic growth and income redistribution. Marginal economic groups would in time "gracefully succumb" to the diffusion of good living, and in the end, only a small residual group of incorrigibles and incompetents would remain. And for these the public dole was available. (Marris & Rein, 1969, p. 10)

In a sense, poverty was not perceived as a part of the social reality during this period of time. Although some governmental agencies, including the Bureau of Census, the Bureau of Labor Statistics, and the Social Security Administration, documented the existence of a large group of American poor, poverty as a public issue did not emerge throughout the 1950s. In fact, it did not become a dominant issue until after the presidential campaign of 1960. Lewis Coser, as noted by Stephen Rose, states:

> Historically, the poor emerge when society elects to recognize poverty as a special status and assigns specific persons to that category. The fact that some people may privately consider themselves poor is sociologically irrelevant. What is sociologically relevant is poverty as a socially recognized condition, as a social status. (Rose, 1970)

A review of the literature indicates that by 1960, through the convergence of a number of forces and events, poverty became relevant as a public policy problem, and several social-historical and economic factors during the 1950s and early 1960s resulted in the assumptions leading to the Community Action Program (CAP). The predominant events, in summary, include: the civil rights movement, in-migration of blacks to northern industrial cities, high unemployment among blacks, the redefinition of poverty, and the rise of Aid to Families with Dependent Children (AFDC) (Naparstek, 1971, 1972).

The Community Mental Health Centers Act of 1963, reviewed earlier in this chapter, was part of a bewildering array of social legislation that was passed by Congress in the 1960s. A review of American social policy from the New Deal to the present indicates that domestic policy had never before been so explicitly selective in programs and services directed towards particular groups of citizens. The litany of new legislation directed at problems of mental health, race, delinquency, urban and rural poverty, unemployment, and physical deterioration of inner cities included, in addition to the Community Mental Health Centers Act, the Area Development Act and the Model Cities programs incorporated in the Demonstration Cities Act.

The 1960s witnessed the federal government becoming explicitly committed to countering poverty and racial discrimination through the utilization of a vast array of social services. Medical services were mistakenly treated as a mere subset of social services. This was reinforced as public and private expenditures for health, education, and welfare services grew more rapidly than the general growth of the economy between 1960 and 1968. S. M. Miller notes that from 10.56% of the gross national product in 1960, services grew to 17.7% in 1964, and 19.8% in 1968. In terms of dollar expenditures, services doubled between 1960 and 1968, with the public sector growing more rapidly than the private (Naparstek, 1972). Martin Rein points out that the emerging prominence of social services was not only because of the expenditure level.

He states,

> The primary factor that thrust the social services into prominence during this period was a reinterpretation of their mission and the unobstrusive inclusion of this new function in diverse types of social legislation directed toward different problems and populations. (Rein, 1970, p. 327)

Distinct conceptual frames of reference appear to have influenced the development of human services and the way in which they subsequently emerged through the War on Poverty. The policy and ideological basis for these programs emerged from the Ford Foundation Grey Areas Project, the President's Committee on Juvenile Delinquency, the Joint Commission on Mental Health and Illness, and the amendments to the 1962 Social Security Act. The Ford Foundation's Grey Areas Project, followed by the President's Committee work, provided the theoretical rationale for the subsequent CAP. This approach to human services represented a significant departure from the traditional view of how services should be delivered. The explanation of poverty offered was that social structural aspects of society were the causes of the problem, and radical reform of the institutions was necessary. The President's Committee came under the influence of Ohlin's and Cloward's "opportunity theory." This theory offered operational suggestions for the elimination of delinquency, but also provided a conceptual focus on mechanisms by which institutions within the social structure perpetuate deviance and poverty (Naparstek, 1971).

The 1962 amendments created a strategy aimed towards helping families become self-supporting, rather than dependent on welfare checks. Ellen Winston notes that these amendments attempted to make public welfare a more constructive instrument to reduce dependency by emphasizing individual rehabilitation through a quasitherapeutic approach (Winston, 1965). The mental health initiative also aimed at reducing dependency by focusing preventive work at the community level. In social work litany, severe mental illness was often treated as though it was another poverty problem. Pluralistic ignorance became public policy.

In late 1969, the entire mental health and social service system was caught up in a web of politics. The White House, through HEW, had established a host of interagency task forces whose mission was to reconceptualize the administration of human services. A summary of task force reports identified the following as longstanding problems: (1) Services were unfocused and lacking in clear priorities; (2) services were forced on persons unwilling to accept them; (3) services were inaccessible to persons wanting and needing them; (4) services were unresponsive to those needs felt most urgently by states, communities, and neighborhoods; and (5) services were fragmented with inadequate accountability and poor quality control.

Under the guise of administrative reform, the first Nixon administration began to dismantle the service reform initiatives of the early 1960s. A working alliance between mental health and human service professionals, social and political scientists, policy analysts, politicans, foundation executives, federal bureaucrats, and others, attempted to force a national effort to master the complexities of social, economic, and regional problems. By the end of the decade, these alliances had broken down and public support for the War on Poverty dramatically abated. Programs originally conceived as selectively oriented toward serving the poor were soon to be perceived with even greater selectivity—as programs for poor blacks (Naparstek, 1972). Support for these programs even diminished among minorities. Tom Wicker, for example, noted that the policies somehow managed to alienate many of the blacks and the poor, as well as white conservatives and members of Congress (Moynihan, 1968). Lee Rainwater claimed that these programs made promises to the black community, and-through a pseudoradical rhetoric, angered and insulted the working class, at the same time delivering no more than symbolic resources to black people (Naparstek, 1972; Rainwater, 1970).

Perhaps the pessimism of Alfred Kahn best summarizes the harsh judgments on what transpired during the 1960s:

> To review the history of service reform initiatives for the early 1960s is to discover that there has been very little effect to reconstruct the basic delivery system, as a system. There has been rhetoric and ideology. Much has been accomplished that has validity in the domains of political and social action and social change. Much has been accomplished elsewhere in the social sector: employment and housing programs, income maintenance, housing. But there has been little systematic learning about this, about organization for personal services—after millions of dollars of service and research investment. In fact, few good questions have been asked. (Kahn, 1974, p. 8)

LOOKING AHEAD

What went wrong? Why did many significant reforms and many important research efforts carried out in the 1960s and 1970s result in such failure? Perhaps more important, where do we go from here? How should mental health and human services be reassessed?

During the past two decades, human problems have been defined, as we have seen, in the context of macrosocial and economic forces. It is our contention that a microanalysis is now needed, addressed on the one hand towards the neighborhood context and on the other hand towards the specific needs of severely ill individuals. This dual approach emphasizes the importance of the individual as a biopsychosocial entity living and interacting in a neighborhood. While this book concentrates on the neighborhood, the authors fully recognize that both forms of microanalysis are required (Naparstek & Haskell, 1977).

At no other time in the history of the United States has America's nongovernmental sector been faced with a greater challenge than at the present time. Social inventions leading to cooperative efforts between public, private, and nonprofit organizations are urgently required. While the needs of people approach the infinite, the resources available are terribly finite. In today's economy and in an era of reduced governmental services and funding, resources are further limited. As a result of inflation, slow economic growth, and the unwillingness of citizens to pay high taxes, public budgets—which in the past supported service delivery operations—are now shrinking. Local financial obligations continue, especially in the older cities where the population consists of large proportions of disadvantaged people; however, aid in the form of grants from federal to local governments is on the downturn, and simultaneously grants from state to local governments are threatened as fiscal limits are reached at the state levels.

Shrinking public resources suggest both opportunities and problems. On one hand, diminishing public funds may result in drastic cutbacks in public service provisions; on the other hand, by limiting the size of the public budget, a new repertoire for services delivery must be developed.

The ability of community groups, self-help, and other nonprofit organizations to meet the multiple challenges of these changing times means increased attention must be paid to building their capacity to cope. New strategies are now needed.

In a review of models and strategies of alternative service delivery, we find that they are numerous and diverse (National Commission on Neighborhoods, 1979a). The following programs and strategies can be identified: Activities include physical improvements in the neighborhoods ("sweat equity" and development), strategies for decentralizing public services, and strategies for deregulation and the modification of laws (i.e., control of investment and disinvestment practices, environmental improvements). Some organizations focus on service delivery— day care, health services, anticrime programs, recreational programs, mental health, or services to selected groups of people. Still other organizations are exclusively involved in development activities—building and rehabilitating housing, transportation, revitalizing commercial strips, building community centers or cultural plazas, and general economic development—that result in increased job opportunities. It is to America's nongovernmental sector that this country must now look for a response to these very serious challenges.

However, a policy framework is needed so that these efforts can be proactive, rather than reactive. Policies are needed to support cooperative planning, to deal with the vulnerabilities of people and neighborhood structures while they are incipient, and to treat them before they become chronic.

The goals of these policies would include a desire for public accountability, efficiency, a pluralistic approach to service delivery, and citizen access to the institution that is delivering the service.

CHAPTER 5

Achieving Human Scale
A Policy Framework for Building Partnerships

Mental health professionals have earnestly sought to bring services into the community arena. Although the community mental health movement has had a profound impact on service delivery, neither providers nor consumers have been satisfied with developments during the past decade. Services tend to be delivered in a fragmented manner. They are often offered in an inefficient, duplicative, and bureaucratically confusing fashion. There is a distinct lack of accountability in the various delivery systems. There is failure to minister to prolonged needs or even to provide comprehensive analysis of clients' problems.

In examining the initiatives that evolved from the Great Society programs and the later Nixon and Ford federalism, we have seen how past national initiatives in the area of human services and mental health have led to a proliferation of federal programs, each with its own set of regulations and channels of funding.

OBSTACLES TO SERVICE: FRAGMENTATION, ACCESSIBILITY, ACCOUNTABILITY

Among the major mental health and human service delivery system problems discussed in the last chapter were fragmentation, lack of accessibility, and lack of accountability. Crosscutting each of these problems is the fact that informal community helping systems are not recognized, not utilized, and do not form an integrated service

This chapter is based on the work of Arthur Naparstek, David Biegel, Chester Haskell, and Wendy Sherman. See: Biegel, 1979, 1982; Naparstek & Biegel, 1982; Naparstek & Haskell, 1981; and Sherman & Haskell, 1980.

resource. Although knowledge exists about neighborhood helping networks, they have never been sufficiently utilized to address the issues of fragmentation and lack of accessibility and accountability. Solutions have been sought in bureaucratic overregulations, rule making, and centralization into burgeoning bureaucracies. These solutions are not only wasteful, expensive, and stultifying to individual effort; they also produce an effect opposite to that intended.

Fragmentation of service programs results partially from our pluralistic service system. Government agencies, sectarian agencies, private nonprofit social service agencies, profit-making agencies, and community helpers all provide various service programs on the neighborhood, city, state, and national levels, with each agency receiving funding from a variety of sources. A single community mental health center may receive money from federal, state, and local governments; from the United Way; from national and local foundations; from fee-for-service; and through grants, contracts, purchase of service, insurance reimbursements, and so forth. The concomitant variety of funding sources, periods, levels, eligibility criteria, regulations, and mechanisms renders the development of a coordinated service delivery network extremely difficult. Superimposing additional "coordinating" bureaucracies compounds the problem—more administrative hierarchies to burn money.

The administrative obstacles cited often lead to wasted and/or misused funds. If, for example, children's services are needed in a given neighborhood, but money for alcoholics is more readily available, usually alcoholics receive services, not children. Then, too, the matter of funding and its availability often involves taking the responsibility for establishing service priorities from the service deliverer, who is closest to the neighborhood needs, and placing them on the city, state, or national level—or worse yet, with elitist "planning agencies," whose board members would never dream of setting foot in the involved neighborhoods or using their programs. Patients, clients, and neighborhoods are forgotten as the institutional imperative reigns supreme.

Fragmentation often occurs because service providers are unaware of the types and amounts of services that are provided in the community by other agencies. They are even less aware of nonprofessional services provided by informal neighborhood helping networks. For instance, our research (Naparstek, Biegel, & Spence, 1979) showed that families were the major locus of problems in the two communities investigated, but that helpers were unable to describe a cohesive service system to serve families. Many helpers were unaware of which service networks were utilized by community residents to address their problems. Agranoff (1977) determined that 40% to 80% of all clients are multiproblem clients. They need services from more than one agency. Lack of information about available services can and does result in inadequate, fragmented, and therefore ineffective help for those in need.

Lack of services is not the sole issue. The National Conference on Social Welfare (1977) recently reported findings and recommendations of a major study of problems in the delivery of social services funded by HEW. Of special interest is documentation of the extraordinary number of social service agencies and programs. Over 300 social programs are made available by HHS alone; the average state has 80 to 100 service programs. There are over 79,000 state and local governments, each administering a variety of service programs for their constituents. The average large city has some 400 to 500 private and government programs and/or agencies. Lack of service integration—even with a multitude of services available—still results in service vacuums. A review of available formal services shows that most are oriented to crisis; there is a severe shortage of preventive services. Trained psychiatrists are a scarce commodity. The severely ill receive a plethora of putative "social services"; in many cases, they do not receive the care of professionals trained to treat specific disorders.

Accessibility obstacles can also prevent people from seeking and receiving help. Among such obstacles are: services that are provided at inconvenient hours and locations; services that are narrowly defined; services that cost too much; services that are delivered in an inappropriate or insensitive manner; services that are poorly designed because they do not account for class and ethnic differences among clients; and the absence of crucial services by trained psychiatrists. Accessibility issues often arise because of legal obstacles such as conflicting eligibility criteria for given services, or because of the multiplicity of funding sources and their requisite spending regulations. Legal obstacles at present also prevent mediating institutions, such as churches, ethnic clubs, or community organizations, from receiving, for example, federal mental health moneys, despite the advantages of access they offer in the development of community-based preventative and rehabilitative programs. The private agencies that receive "contract" money are often city-wide organizations with highly skilled "lobbying" executives, but no real neighborhood roots. Lack of awareness of helping resources by service providers limits their ability to refer, or to martial together, a number of resources for multiproblem clients. In fact, Naparstek, Biegel, and Spence (1979) found that helpers of all kinds are unaware of resources outside of their own sphere or interest, and those resources that they name most frequently present few choices for people in need.

Accountability is an important element of service delivery because interactive relationships are necessary between the individuals being served and the service decision makers, in order to ensure that clients can influence decisions that affect them and to promote sensitivity to their needs and interests (Gilbert, 1973). Agranoff (1977) points out that services often lack such interactive relationships and that this causes severe accountability problems. For example, despite the important helping services being provided by community helpers who have first-hand knowledge of problems and concerns of people on the neighborhood level, professional agencies often do not understand or respect the role that community helpers already play or could play on behalf of individual clients. These helpers are allowed little input into agency planning, service delivery, and evaluation processes.

Finally, it is increasingly clear that no single sector of the mental health or human service system has the resources—fiscal, political, administrative, legal, or personal—to effect, by itself, these problems of fragmentation and lack of accessibility and accountability. To further complicate matters, there is the problem of categorical programming, which is often cited as the creator of these difficulties. Yet categorical programs were a response to the legitimate needs of interest groups representing high-risk population groups, including neglected and abused children, youth, the elderly, handicapped, and disabled, welfare recipients, and minorities, among others. The real needs of these different target populations still exist and must be taken into account.

GETTING SERVICES TO PEOPLE

An entirely new perspective for getting services to people is needed. With all its imperfections—and all its promise—the Community Mental Health Empowerment Process approach, tested in Baltimore, Maryland, and Milwaukee, Wisconsin, is such an approach. This approach takes into account the diversity, individuality, and potential of city people in neighborhoods. It is based on assumptions that lead to a new way of involving people in the process of giving and receiving help. New dimensions of citizen participation are advocated. The process focuses on the unique strengths and helping resources of neighborhoods, and it builds on these resources to create partnerships between community and professional helping networks (see chapters 6 and 7).

As noted in the Task Panel Report to the President's Commission on Mental Health:

> Mental health services should be offered to individuals first on their assets and strengths, maintaining and cultivating their membership in social networks and natural communities in the least restructive environment. This would mean developing methods which could identify and assess the functioning of an individual's natural support system, and establishing, where appropriate, linkages between the natural support systems and the professional caregiving systems based on a respect for privacy and on genuine cooperation and collaboration, not cooptation and control. . . . Helping people where they are and assisting them to help themselves allows entry into the help giving and receiving system without requiring that a person be labeled "patient" or deemed "sick." (1978, Vol. 2, p. 154)

Our intent is not to define a social policy framework that will be cased exclusively in policy and program terms. Rather, we are striving to develop policy initiatives to support a pluralistic process that requires involvement from all concerned sectors in a city and can meet the diverse needs of different groups of people. There is no help to be found in dealing with mental health issues in a blender that neither distinguishes the variety of individual problems nor recognizes the spectrum of individual neighborhood resources.

ESSENTIAL PARTNERSHIPS

It has finally dawned on America, the land of plenty, that its resources—natural and human—might not be endless. As budgets are tightening, demands are increasing for cost-effectiveness to meet society's needs. One approach has been the call for partnerships. President Carter's urban policy message of 1979 called for the development of partnerships among all sectors—local, state, and federal government, business and the private sector, the voluntary sector, and the neighborhood—as a necessary process for solving the complex problems faced by urban and rural communities alike. While such partnerships already exist in some cases, they are neither automatic nor obvious. The remainder of this chapter is designed to assist the mental health practitioner in understanding the prerequisites for developing partnerships and the means for achieving those partnerships.

The central prerequisite for partnerships is that *all* relevant actors, whether they are mental health professionals, human service administrators, or community representatives, must be able to interact with one another effectively. Appropriate partnerships presuppose the achievement of a mutual respect among all partners and acknowledgment of differing skills and experiences. Even in working multi-party groups, such relationships are rare. Thus, a critical ingredient of any approach to building partnerships must be the creation of means for enabling and encouraging such reciprocal relationships among diverse, and often competing, parties.

Another crucial factor is that the partnerships that are desired must, of necessity, be locality-based because their objectives are related to a specific neighborhood or subsection of a city. This does not mean that the locality is the only perspective, but that the neighborhood ought to be both the locus and focus of the partnership. The nature of the particular neighborhood, its residents, its relationship with city government, and a host of other variables will mean that the capacities of actors to fulfill partnership roles—to play their parts—are likely to be highly varied. Simultaneously, the specific needs of individual neighborhoods will vary.

Given such complexities, what must be done to promote partnerships? First, there must be a recognition of the need to build individual and organizational capacity to play partnership roles. The key is making certain that each actor has the wherewithal—however appropriate or defined—to fill his/her partnership role effectively. Given the fact that different neighborhoods have different needs, there are numerous modes of fostering these abilities. These range from provision of technical assistance, to increase the bookkeeping and managerial skills in a community organization, to hiring experts with sophisticated human service expertise; from instruction in individual community and groups skills to obtaining consultation by policy analysts. On the one hand, there simply may be a need for some seed money to hire professional staff; on the other, a package of technical assistance and personnel to put together a mental health program. The point is that the range of possibilities is as broad as the range of neighborhood problems and situations.

Community organizations are not the only institutions in need of some means of increasing their capabilities to perform in such partnership roles. Many of the problems of partnerships arise because public officials, both elected and appointed, as well as people of the private sector, lack the skills required in successful working partnerships.

Recognizing the evident need for formulation of such partnerships carries with it no guarantee they will, in fact, occur. The major precondition of any partnership—the requirement for mutual respect and acknowledgment of needed diverse skills among partners—is rarely achieved. Rather, local government agencies hold most of "the cards" and neighborhood organizations must either play by the city or state's rules or force the attention of the city through the politics of confrontation. This situation is both an issue of the political process and an issue of structure.

THE SPECIAL GENIUS OF THE NEIGHBORHOOD

As we discuss partnerships and their potential effectiveness in solving problems we must once again clarify the assumptions from which the basic concept arises. One set of assumptions is about neighborhoods themselves. We assert that neighborhoods are indeed the building blocks of the cities; that people identify with the neighborhoods in which they live. A city is usually an aggregation of neighborhoods since one of the most distinguishing characteristics of large human groups is their diversity. The idea of what constitutes a neighborhood varies from city to city, and even from neighborhood to neighborhood within a city. As we have come to understand the nature of rural communities and neighborhoods and the different situations they face, we have increased awareness of the diversity of neighborhoods. A neighborhood is a self-defining concept. The only people who really know what their neighborhood is are the residents. Neighborhoods are dynamic, alive, and changing places that evolve as people grow older and come and go in the locality. Finally, for any given individual, the concept of neighborhood will vary from day to day and issue to issue. Neighborhood should be regarded, therefore, as being in a constant state of flux.

Another set of assumptions has to do with neighborhood organizations. Like the neighborhoods they spring from, such groups are diverse, changing, and difficult to define. They range from block organizations that have coalesced around a particular, immediate issue, to large, complex, multipurpose corporations that are engaged in the delivery of human services, sophisticated economic development programs, and high-powered political activities. Ideologically, they range from the kinds of groups seeking to build through partnership and cooperation to those concentrating on adversary power politics. The foremost assumption, however, is that a "successful" organization (as defined by the neighborhood it serves) is a positive force for the overall economic and social vitality of that neighborhood.

Neighborhood organizations throughout the nation are performing an amazingly broad range of functions, including the direct provisions of public services (sometimes under contract from local government) in such areas as mental health and health care, services for the elderly, youth activities, drug abuse control projects, housing rehabilitation, and anticrime programs. Some organizations work with local government in undertaking economic and commercial development projects, many on an impressively large scale. Others contribute input into various formal and informal planning processes and citizen participation activities. Some work with local lenders to develop and implement antiredlining programs and to build neighborhood housing. Additional organizations conduct a range of volunteer programs, art projects, religious and ethnic activities, conservation efforts, a wide range of research and demonstration projects, job programs, and historic preservation. Lastly, and perhaps most importantly, neighborhood organizations exert a range of political powers that help—or force—local governments to see things from the neighborhood perspective. Neighborhood organizations also serve often as centers of the political and social activity of their communities.

Besides being a place where people reside, the neighborhood is also a place where they *live*. At its best, it is a place of support, where people feel a sense of belonging. It has familiar comforts, a setting where people can work and relax, where they can raise children and live secure in the knowledge that they have a place in the world. It can be a refuge from the chaos of the urban environment. It is a place of intimacy amid the impersonal metropolis. For these reasons and many more, there has been a deep concern not only with protecting neighborhoods, but also with promoting their growth and revitalization.

BUILDING ON STRENGTHS

One of the chief shortcomings of most federal programs has been the failure to base mental health, human services, and community and economic development initiatives on the strengths, resources, and diversities existing in local communities. Community organizations and organizational and cultural networks that have the capacity to support people in need are bypassed. The neighborhood is rarely linked effectively with the service delivery system.

The process of forming partnerships can serve to expand and revitalize services at a time when no single budget is large enough to meet needs. Such efforts in the neighborhood cannot substitute for planning and services appropriate to city, state, or federal levels. What does take place in the neighborhood, however, is the building and rebuilding of natural support systems, which are both a long-neglected resource and an effective mode of prevention of urban problems. Naparstek (1976), Doughton (1976), and Berger and Neuhaus (1977), among others, argue that people need to feel that daily life is on a manageable and human scale. For most people, that translates into the neighborhood scale, however the people define it. These authors stress the importance of locality-relevant instructions—family, church, neighborhood associations, civic and voluntary associations—which mediate between the private world of the individual and public world of the system. They argue that people working in small groups around concerns of the neighborhood strengthen their internal networks and make it possible to link with other systems for mutual problem-solving.

People tend to determine their resource needs quite subjectively. They are guided by interrelated principles of equity, security, and sufficiency. Citizens must feel that their investment equals their return; that they are economically, physically, and socially secure; and that they have the sufficiency to participate in government, to deal successfully with the problems of their community, exercising some control over institutions that impact directly on their lives.

The degree to which people feel sufficient is often determined by how a neighborhood defines itself and how others define it. People in neighborhoods, then, with a sense of who they are and a feeling of capacity and competence, have the greatest ability to deal with the problems. When people have a sense of their own efficacy, their investment in their community creates psychological, social, and physical supports leading to a healthier individual, family, and neighborhood (Naparstek & Haskell, 1977).

FOSTERING NEIGHBORHOOD CAPACITY FOR URBAN PARTNERSHIPS

Partnerships are meaningless fictions if real people in real communities are unable to cope with their environment. People must have a certain sense of sufficiency in working on their problems. This means one must discuss capacity and how to build it. Neighborhoods throughout the country have varying levels of skill and economic resources, and diverse types of human groupings and networks. Thus it is logical that each neighborhood develops a unique array of needs. To build the capacity for new urban partnerships, cooperation among the professions, government, and neighborhoods is required. Without the capacity to fight for political decisions with skill and power, one enters into a partnership from a position of weakness. Andrew Mott, of the Center for Community Change, commented: "It is difficult to conceive of a true partnership in which one partner has a stranglehold on the resources which are crucial to the other party's ability to function" (National Commission on Neighborhoods, 1979a, p. 355). Without rough equity among partners in terms of either power or resources, programs and projects are doomed to failure. Increasing the capability of all partners to play partnership roles requires a process of capacity building. This requirement applies equally to public officials, businessmen, and citizens. Different types of assistance may be required for each actor. A primary concern must be to target development assistance to meet the requirements of the specific individual, organization and/or neighborhood at a specific point in time.

Steps in the building of the capacity to engage in partnerships include:

1. Enabling all actors to understand the service delivery system within which they operate.
2. Understanding and addressing the existence of fiscal, legal, and administrative obstacles or disincentives.
3. Movement of people away from zero-sum, confrontation (the "us" versus "them" syndrome) to an emphasis on interrelationships.
4. Helping citizens and neighborhood organizations develop the technical and administrative skills required to operate in a decentralized system. This includes resolution of questions of funding.
5. Enabling citizens and public officials to build on the existing networks or organizations and institutions that are the infrastructure of any neighborhood. (Of special interest here are the concepts of "mediating institutions" discussed by Berger and Neuhaus, 1977, and the locality-relevant support systems discussed by Biegel and Naparstek, 1979.)
6. Helping all involved to recognize that empowerment of people and neighborhood revitalization go hand-in-hand.
7. Helping all involved to recognize that each sector brings strengths, as well as weaknesses, to any partnership.

Every potential partnership will be faced with the necessity to cope with a range of tasks in order to develop into an active, problem-solving process. First, each partner, independent of the others, must be able to mobilize its own resources and knowledge. To make sure each sector is "up to speed," technical assistance, the funding of capacity building, and experience are required in support of specific programs, as well as support for the ongoing institutions and individuals involved.

Second, each partner must develop the ability to perform cooperatively concerning both specific problems and an ongoing process. This requires the development of a range of substantive and interpersonal skills. All too often, programs designed to provide support for various revitalization efforts deal only with certain types of needs—those met through technical skills or expertise. What is often forgotten is that working with people requires more than technical knowledge. More important is the human ability to work together, to be able to utilize interpersonal, process-oriented talents. The core of a partnership is not expertise or objective data. What is essential is a capacity to interact mutually in moving towards common goals.

Third, the composition and needs of the partnership and its members will change over time, thus a continuous process of capacity building and support is required. This is especially true in terms of the need to target partnership efforts in particular areas, since neighborhoods and their problems are hardly static. The same is also true for local government and the private sector.

All forms of capacity building must have multiple objectives. On one level, such efforts foster the solution of real problems by increasing the ability of each actor to fulfill his or her appropriate role. Simultaneously, the active interact with other members of a partnership. On a third plane, the process of building formal and informal systems and networks of communication continues.

Ideally, the objectives of capacity building efforts in relation to neighborhoods will include the following:

1. *Equity.* All individuals and groups needing services should have access to them. With limited resources, choices must be made in allocating these resources. Equity requires that priority in resource allocation go to those most in need, least able to afford the services, and most likely to benefit from the services.
2. *Accountability.* Accountability is not a one-way street; the public sector alone should not determine which services are to be delivered to a neighborhood and whether they are delivered appropriately and effectively. Procedures for ensuring dual accountability are necessary. Only if consumers are accountable to providers, and providers are accountable to consumers, can one assure the relevance of the system. Without procedures for dual accountability, we often find providers unable to identify the strengths and needs of an individual and his family. A delivery system cannot be effective if whole individuals are viewed only in relation to separate programs. By building dual accountability procedures into the system, consumers are given an opportunity to express their views and to make those views

count. Thus citizens have a major role in the development of the mental health service from the planning through the evaluation stage.

3. *Accessibility.* Accessibility issues are multidimensional. There are objective and subjective elements. Objective elements include convenient location within the neighborhood, transportation to and from services, and convenient times such as evenings and weekends. Subjective characteristics include flexibility, identity, and empathy. *Flexibility* in the delivery system suggests the pluralistic approach in which economic, social, and cultural differences are taken into account. The notion that different groups of people deal with a crisis and problems differently is given a high priority. *Identity* suggests that the program be designed to reinforce people's positive view of themselves. Through the neighborhood approach, the delivery system will preserve a sense of human scale instead of causing consumers to feel like cogs in an impersonal machine. Building onto the natural helping networks in a neighborhood also assures empathy between professional mental health practitioners and consumers. By linking helping networks to service agencies, it is likely that personnel will be more able to develop the capacity to identify with the aspirations and problems of the consumer.

By joining together different people with different backgrounds to work on one problem of concern, a spirit of cooperation can be engendered. As the team grows and people experience each other, the advantages of mobilizing and employing different perspectives and skills may become obvious. Partners see that they are capable of solving problems as a group and affecting the neighborhood and institutions involved. At the same time, they learn and grow personally, coming to understand the value of cooperation and communication with others. Over time, success breeds success. Every time a partnership successfully deals with a problem in this fashion, the opportunities for personal growth, confidence, and satisfaction are increased.

ASSESSING REALITIES

Finally, the partnership approach compels the tailoring of any capacity-building or technical-assistance effort to deal with realities. Real people who wish to deal with real problems are loathe to invest time in purely theoretical exercises. Any attempt to build a partnership in a particular setting must take into account a host of variables relevant to the situation. Partnerships do not just occur. They require a great deal of hard work by everyone involved. Therefore, any such effort must account for at least six major variables.

1. *People.* Who are the people involved? What are their backgrounds, positions, goals, and values? Under what constraints do they operate?
2. *Needs.* What are their training and technical assistance needs, seen from their own perspective as well as that of others?
3. *Policy.* What are the formal and informal policies, rules, and methods of getting things done?
4. *Problems.* What are the major problems facing each of the actors? Which problems are seen as common and which are peculiar to each other?
5. *Skills.* What competencies does each actor bring to the partnership? What weaknesses? Where are there deficiencies that must be overcome before the partnership can operate?
6. *History.* What has happened in the past that colors each actor's outlook on the problem and on the other actors?

There are three levels of capacity building. The first is development of the individual partner's capability to be able to perform partnership functions. Such development is primarily unilateral and is directed at any of the partners. For neighborhood organizations, this may mean staff and governing board training, establishment of adequate financial accounting systems, the hiring of experienced community development specialists, or a whole host of other possibilities.

The second is the development of interactive, ongoing local problem-solving partnerships. As noted above, this multilateral effort is the central point of any partnership strategy, focusing as it does on cooperation, teamwork, and mutual assistance in the quest for resolution of common local problems. Again, there is a broad range of potential approaches, including the provision of external, group process facilitators, the funding of partnership staff or technical support, and the building of common data bases. While most current programs that support local partnership are limited to one- or two-issue areas such as counseling services or health care, the crucial factor is that the emphasis in partnership building is the development of tactics, mechanisms, patterns of behavior, or political processes that are internal in nature. The focus is intergroup.

FROM PARTNERSHIPS TO NETWORKS

The third level is the development of interpartnership networks. Once the local partnership is formed and has begun an ongoing process of problem solving, it can begin to interact beyond its boundaries. However, it is important to note that the other steps of partner development and partnership building must come first. Locality-based partnerships can only deal with larger, more comprehensive partnerships when they "have their own act together." In other words, the local partnerships precede the network. Another implication of this approach is that local partners will build a sense of community and shared goals among themselves, thus facilitating their interaction as a unit with local partnerships, city-wide organizations, and county, state, and federal government. This approach explicitly recognizes that many neighborhood problems cannot be resolved with a strictly local focus.

A POLICY CONTEXT FOR THE NEIGHBORHOOD APPROACH TO CAPACITY BUILDING

The partnership building process is one that needs to be supported by policies at different levels of government. First, policy makers must analyze existing policies to eliminate unintended discouragement of local capacity building. Public officials who have not accurately assessed the local environment may create unintended consequences by increasing paperwork and/or putting forth rules and regulations that become legal and administrative obstacles to change. Area-wide boards and civil service bureaucracies may discourage neighborhood initiatives.

Second, policy makers need to develop programs that are flexible. If policy makers cannot develop greater flexibility, we may continue to perpetuate what is often called "grant junkeyship." This means that neighborhood groups, towns, and cities will define their needs in terms of federal and state priorities, whether or not these are real needs of the community. Such a process only reinforces mutual suspicion on all sides that people are applying for funds inappropriately or spending those funds in ways that were unintended in the legislation. Folks only think that because it is true! Such a process also undermines accurate analysis of a problem since it encourages citizens and cities to seek the solution in such a way that it matches up with a predetermined problem and categorical funding source. State funding bureaucracies that ignore rural, urban, and suburban differences are the worst offenders.

Third, policies are needed that create incentives for building partnerships at the local level. Two approaches are required for such an incentive system. In one instance, funding needs to be available not only to the community sectors, but also to consortiums or partnerships of the public and private sectors. Such funding programs might initially be only small seed moneys to meet specific goals of a beginning partnership. Although government would certainly need to know how funds are being spent, such funding might be available to a consortium rather than to an incorporated group. Or one sector might act as lead partner, offering its accounting and staff services to meet government regulations. In another instance, government can encourage partnerships by implementing a concept of mutual concurrence. For example, in some federal programs, mayors must concur with a neighborhood group's proposed activity; in instances where a city program is going into a neighborhood, neighborhood groups should also be required to concur.

Fourth, policies are needed to increase funding for capacity-building training and technical assistance for partnerships at the local level. Both the Task Panel on Community Support Systems of the President's Commission on Mental Health (1978) and the Final Report of the National Commission on Neighborhoods (1979b) recommended a number of policy initiatives that are supportive of the partnership notion.

PITFALLS OF TOP-DOWN POLICY MAKING

The experiences of the 1960s and 1970s suggest that policy makers and politicians still have a tendency to respond to complex human problems with dramatic, but simplistic, top-down remedies. More often than not, the more grandiose the scheme, the messier the unintended consequence.

Thus, we can assume that the decentralization of services and a straight resource approach to neighborhoods, by themselves, will not support a viable neighborhood climate. Although the community mental health movement was predicated on the notion that its programs could improve the overall quality of community life, little attention has been given by mental health professionals to the complex set of legal, administrative, and fiscal policies that independently and/or collectively make it difficult or impossible to bring about change. These are obstacles to change that are structured into the urban system and act to create a set of disincentives for neighborhood viability. For example, neighborhoods cannot maintain a viable infrastructure (network) if local and state policies, ordinances, regulations, and judicial decisions negatively impact on a community. Furthermore, such public actions often serve as legal obstacles that inhibit participation and foster a sense of insufficiency among residents. Another example is the relationship between general municipal services and neighborhood approaches to the human services. Interdependence among the delivery systems for various types of services is essential to a healthy community environment. The inequitable distribution of city services stimulates conditions in which people will not stay in a given neighborhood. Such disincentives serve to break down neighborhood-based networks and thus permit and engender conditions of inequity and insufficiency. Thus, a primary precondition for change must be the identification of such disincentives, their removal, and the concomitant creation of incentives for the maintenance and enhancement of neighborhood-based networks.

The decisions facing local mental health professionals on neighborhood-related issues are complex and politically hazardous. Often practitioners are confronted with a dwindling tax base, aging housing stock, increased numbers of aged and dependent people, underemployment, and a breakdown in social service delivery systems. All these elements lead to varied conditions of alienation and make it difficult to decentralize services in any meaningful way.

Mental health legislation needs to be enacted in order to facilitate a comprehensive approach towards restructuring the processes of governance through a mixture of centralization and decentralization of public and private service delivery systems. Legislation also needs to be developed to eliminate systemic origins of neighborhood decline. Perhaps the greatest challenge confronting community psychiatry and the entire field of human services is to meld federal funds and programs with local conditions in ways that will increase utilization of services and decrease racial and other out-group tension and polarizations.

PART TWO

The second major section of this volume is, in essence, a detailed report on the evolution of a model process for conceiving, planning, and delivering appropriate mental health services at the neighborhood level— and on a human scale. In the course of our analysis of what happened over the four years of the Neighborhood and Family Services Project, which the National Institute of Mental Health funded in South East Baltimore, Maryland, and the Southside of Milwaukee, Wisconsin, we shall continue to argue for the advantages of the approach epitomized by the project and advocated in preceding pages. Yet it must be stressed that what was developed in both neighborhoods was not the result of preconceived notions of suitable mental health programming that the authors and their colleagues exported to the two neighborhoods.

The intent of the project from the beginning was to generate a process through which residents of the two communities would, themselves, assess their own mental health needs, then identify and capitalize on their inherent strengths and resources to put into place an array of programs that they deemed appropriate. Implicit in developing the capacity to undertake and direct such programs would be the forging of links and then partnerships among community people, professionals working in the field of mental health, informal helpers working in the neighborhood, and various political and funding entities within and outside the neighborhood.

Ownership of the project and resultant programs was always invested in the community itself and always perceived by everyone concerned to be invested in the community—never in the University of Southern California, the initiating entity; never in the professionals who were hired to carry out policies or staff programs. The project was the community's own "baby." Recognition of this fact is essential to an understanding of what happened—and is still happening—in South East Baltimore and Southside Milwaukee, and to an appreciation of what can be learned from developments there.

Thus, in the pages that follow, when occasional references are made to "our" project, this is something of a misnomer. For while the authors invested time, energy, and professional resources in the project, and held high expectations for it, it really should not be regarded as "ours." The project and the credit for its success belonged to—and still belongs to—the people of South East Baltimore and Southside Milwaukee. They made it their project. They made it work.

All of this was just the way it was supposed to be. Which is why the project strikes us as well worth reporting, studying, and perhaps emulating. Recommendations for public policy initiatives, which might enable other communities around the United States to adapt the Neighborhood Mental Health Empowerment Process to their own needs in both mental health and human services, follow our report on the specifics of the project.

Preliminary Assumptions and Principles

The Community Mental Health Empowerment Model is based on a framework of assumptions and principles supported by a significant body of literature. Research outlined in this chapter touches upon issues of social class, ethnicity, and mental health; underserved and inadequately served population groups; community support systems; competency and power; and community and professional roles. While it is not intended to be a review of all pertinent literature in these areas, the summary here demonstrates that the assumptions underlying the authors' model are logically based on previous work.

ASSUMPTION 1

Social class and ethnicity are significant variables that affect attitudes towards, and use of, mental health services. The bridge between research findings and program development appears unconstructed. Class and ethnic differences have often been neglected in the design of mental health service delivery systems. Monolithic models developed in Washington or remote state capitols all too often are aimed at a theoretical lowest common denominator.

Among those who have studied the interrelationship between social class and mental health are Hollingshead and Redlich (1958), Gurin, Veroff, and Feld (1960), Srole and Fischer, (1962), and Myers and Bean (1968). The pioneering work of Hollingshead and Redlich, using the Veterans Administration Diagnostic Classification as a measure of

This chapter is based in part on D. Biegel, *Help-seeking and Receiving in Urban Ethnic neighborhoods.* Unpublished doctoral dissertation, University of Maryland, 1982.

mental illness, and Hollingshead's Index of Social Position as a measure of social class, determined that each social class exhibited distinct types of mental illness among its members; and that the treatment of psychiatric patients within the various classes differed accordingly. The lower the social class, the higher the rates of psychoses and the lower the rates of neuroses. The lower the class, the more likely the patient would be to receive hospital care and the less likely that he would receive outpatient treatment. Siassi, Crocetti, and Spiro (1976) confirmed that this latter phenomenon still occurred 20 years after the Hollingshead–Redlich studies and held true in all areas served by community mental health centers.

Studies by Srole and Fischer, by Myers and Bean, and by Gurin *et al.* support these findings. Gurin's 1960 study was part of a large national mental health survey by the Joint Commission on Mental Illness and Health, which paved the way for the Community Mental Health Centers Act of 1963. Like Hollingshead and Redlich, Gurin found a low utilization of psychiatric help by persons of the lower classes. The Gurin study determined that the lack of help-seeking among the poor did not stem from the lack of distress or motivation, but rather from their frequent encounters with greater economic, educational, and treatment barriers. The poor made less active use of their own resources (family and friends), other professional resources (such as physicians), and informal resources (clergy, community leaders, etc.). They exhibited more passive attitudes towards help-seeking.

Myers and Bean (1968), in their follow-up of 1,563 patients interviewed by Hollingshead and Redlich, explored three hypotheses: (1) that social class affects treatment outcome; (2) that social class affects rehospitalization; and (3) that social class affects adjustment in the community. Their findings indicated that the lower the social class, the lower the likelihood of recovery, the higher the chances of rehospitalization, and the lower the likelihood of adjustment in the community.

The correlation between mental health and social class, then, is well documented. The poor clearly run a high risk of experiencing mental illness, which may prove catastrophic for both patients and families. If hospitalized, chances are meager for a return to the community. If discharged or treated at an outpatient clinic, the impact of mental illness is maximal, resulting in serious employment and financial problems and a high degree of social isolation.

Spiro and his associates (Spiro, Crocetti, Siassi, Ward, & Hansen, 1975; Spiro, Siassi, & Crocetti, 1975a, b) in a series of epidemiologic and utilization studies of blue-collar workers, demonstrated that these workers have rates of mental illness comparable to the population at large, but underutilized services and were more likely to be hospitalized when ill. Moreover, the long-term consequence of even curable, moderate illness was often disastrous downward social mobility and chronicity. Special blue-collar programs had a demonstrated value in modifying these patterns.

The assumption of a relationship between mental health and ethnicity is drawn from the work of anthropologists Mead, Benedict and Kluckholm, as well as from psychiatrists Sullivan, Horney, Ferenezi and Kardiner, all of whom stressed the influence of social and cultural environment in normal and deviant people (Giordano, 1973). Through a review of literature on ethnicity and mental health, Giordano concluded that ethnicity has at least as powerful an influence on mental health as socioeconomic status because ethnicity influences "identity," which in turn influences an individual's mental health:

> The search for identity is a basic psychological need, and ethnicity is a powerful and subtle influence in determining its shape and form. Yet many social scientists have tended to view identity only as a "crisis" or a state of "confusion." In doing so they have neglected the healthy aspect of identification that leads to greater development of self-esteem, group solidarity, and mechanisms to cope with stress. (Giordano, 1973, p. 10)

Giordano refocused attention on the relationship between ethnicity and mental health. His review of early epidemiological studies on the incidence and prevalence of psychiatric disorders in the United States in the 1940s and 1950s suggests a strong link between ethnicity and physical and emotional disorders. He believes that the influence of cultural norms and standards on mental health and mental illness needs more attention.

Opler (1967) has examined early empirical research measuring the effects of ethnicity on mental and physical health. He reports that Haven Emerson found ethnic differences in a prevalence of measles, diptheria, and scarlet fever rates in a 1913 study. In New York State, M. Calabresi found varying occurrences of diabetes, heart disease, pneumonia, and tuberculosis among persons of Italian, Irish, German, Polish, and British extraction. According to Opler and Klopfer in the *Psychiatric Quarterly* of 1944, and Malzberg, even earlier, found differing frequencies in major mental illness among such groups as Italian, Irish, and German immigrants. In 1944, R. W. Hyde and associates also found striking variations in Selective Service rejectees from the Boston area in a study of persons of Chinese, Irish, Italian, Jewish, and Portuguese derivation. Subjects were compared for incidence of psychoses, neuroses, mental deficiency, psychopathic personality, and chronic alcoholism. An underlying assumption of Opler's review was the argument that a person's experiences are structured and interpreted by his culture. Building on the work of Sullivan, Deithelm, Hill, Fromm-Reichmann, and others in the field of psychotherapy of the schizophrenias, Opler argued that interpersonal relations and stresses implicit in various cultures shape manifestations of the disease processes. Cultural issues may define the type, scope, and direction of treatment of mental illness.

Ethnic differences may also be significantly associated with mental health because of their influence upon family relations, role orientations, responses to pain, and use of appropriate mental health resources. Barrabe and Von Mering (1953), in "Ethnic Variation in Mental Stress in Families with Psychotic Children," examined 69 Italian, Jewish, and old American families. They determined that membership in certain ethnic groups could become a source of stress because ethnic values influenced family relations significantly. Results from their study showed, for example, significant differences in the mother–son relationship according to ethnic background. Spiegel (1965), scrutinizing societal responses to social welfare needs and problems, observed variations in basic values among American, Italian, and Irish working-class families. Once again, because ethnic groups were shown to define family roles differently, role conflict within the family might arise and create different stresses.

Zborowski (1964) did a cross-cultural examination of responses to pain among patients of Jewish, Italian, Irish, and old American origins. He found that responses to pain are learned and patterned as part of the individual's culture, and that different ethnic groups respond to pain differently. Fandetti and Gelfand (1978) conducted research on attitudes towards psychiatric symptoms and services in Polish and Italian neighborhoods in Baltimore and compared their findings to those of the Dohrenwends (1976), who studied Irish, Jews, blacks, and Puerto Ricans. Their data suggest that there are differential perceptions of appropriate mental health resources among disparate ethnic groups in American society.

Ethnicity exerts a powerful influence on mental health and mental illness, as does social class. Whereas many mental health professionals accept the effects of socioeconomic differences, there tends to be a certain denial of ethnic variations. This may reflect the inability to replace American "melting-pot" folklore with the realities of cultural pluralism today.

The cry to return psychiatry exclusively to "mainstream" medicine (often translated as somatic medicine) is built on the myth that medical disorders exist in isolation from a social and ethnic context. The mythology itself may require understanding.

Why do some professionals persist in an either-or approach? Somatic contributing factors are obviously very crucial for major psychiatric illnesses. Does this mean that earlier studies of social class and ethnicity were in error? The fact that the tubercle bacillus "causes" tuberculosis has not deterred those concerned with tuberculosis control from attending to strong evidence concerning the effects of socioeconomic status, life circumstances, and ethnicity on tuberculosis spread and control. Are there countertransference issues among key professionals who deny their own socioeconomic and ethnic roots? Has the price of upward mobility and mainstream assimilation efforts been selective inattention to patients' cultural and class issues? Has the dominant cultural value of the supremacy of technology blinded us to the obvious? Among multiply caused disorders, there is no contradiction between studies about sociocultural contributing factors and somatic contributing factors. Ignorance of the one is no more justifiable than ignorance of the other.

This first "assumption," that sociocultural variables are of importance in systems design, is well documented by three decades of research. It is a big assumption in the programs described in this volume, not as a substitute for understanding of somatic variables, but as a vital additional variable in understanding multiply caused mental dysfunctions.

ASSUMPTION 2

The mental health system, striving to build a nationwide network of mental health services, has failed to take into account the nature of America's pluralistic society in which people meet needs and solve problems in varying ways. As a result, current mental health services either fail to serve or are underutilized by such groups as the white working class, racial minorities, the elderly, and women.

THE WORKING CLASS

The underutilization of mental health services by the working class has been documented by Hollingshead and Redlich, and by Gurin. Other studies of note are by Spiro and his colleagues (1975; 1975a, b), Giordano (1973; Giordano & Giordano, 1976), and Brown (1976). Giordano (1973) states that the lower-middle-class white ethnic has tended to avoid public welfare and mental health services because of the special stigma attached to mental illness. He feels that the label "client" or "patient" that has been attached to mental health services has carried with it a stigma that the lower-middle-class white ethnic has tried to avoid.

Bertram Brown, former Director of the National Institute of Mental Health, reported in 1975 on an NIMH-funded study by Glasser, Duggan, and Hoffman, begun in 1970, that documented the low usage of mental health services by United Auto Workers Union members. The researchers found that three principal obstacles accounted for the low utilization of services by UAW union workers:

1. Little knowledge of services—only 13% of the UAW union members knew of mental health coverage in their union contracts.
2. Referral agents—persons most likely to be in a position to make referrals did not do so because they felt workers would not go for help.
3. Workers' reluctance to recognize or discuss their problems.

Spiro, Crocetti, Siassi, Ward, and Hansen, (1975) and Spiro, Siassi, and Crocetti, (1975a, b) reported the results of a series of studies with the UAW union workers in Baltimore aimed at overcoming those obstacles. They confirmed Glasser's findings in two different replication studies. Then, using union officials on an advisory board and union counselors and shop stewards as indigenous workers, they developed a model Labor Union Clinic through which they were able to increase utilization of services significantly and to reach people in need earlier in their illness. Hospitalization rates and long-term disability were both reduced by these programs.

BLACKS

The President's Commission on Mental Health (1978) states that much of what has been known about racial minorities until recently was drawn from the studies that focused on the urban ghettos (e.g., Lewis, 1961; Liebow, 1976; Moynihan, 1965; Rainwater, 1966). Most of these studies did not deal directly with questions of mental health. The relationships among race, mental health, and utilization of services have been described by Carter (1973), Thomas and Sillen (1972), Grier and Cobbs (1968), Bradshaw (1977), and the President's Commission on

Mental Health (1978). All demonstrate that racial differences are a very significant factor in the utilization of mental health services.

The President's Commission on Mental Health (1978) observed that the rate of institutionalization among blacks is about 40% higher than among whites. During the past few decades, this rate has increased among blacks and decreased among whites. Blacks are not only more likely to be institutionalized, but also twice as likely to suffer fatal consequences of mental illness.

Recently, mental health professionals have begun to accept the fact that many of the older models of mental health practice may not be applicable to black communities. Thomas and Comer (1973), for example, pointed out that the mental health of blacks must be viewed within the context of total culture and societal systems, as well as within the perspective of the black groups. Wilcox (1973) suggested that the mental health problems of blacks are compounded by reactions and adaptations to the living conditions and institutional pressures of being a racial minority.

Thus, blacks are not only at a higher risk of experiencing mental illness, but also are less likely to return to normal community life. This problem is intensified by the unwillingness of society to address this issue on a sustained, consistent basis. (See, e.g., Congressional Budget Office, 1977; President's Commission on Mental Health, 1978; Sue, McKinney, Allen, & Hall, 1974.)

HISPANICS

The 1970 census identified Hispanic-Americans as one of the most rapidly growing racial minorities in the United States. The 1975 Current Population Reports estimated that there are at least 11.2 million Hispanics in the United States. Even by the most conservative estimates, the number of Hispanics in the United States is likely to become larger than the number of blacks within a decade or so (Macias, 1977). There have been some studies focusing on the mental health of blacks, but knowledge about the mental health of Hispanics is even more limited.

Padilla and Ruiz (1973) and Padilla, Ruiz, and Alvarez (1975) have documented that Hispanics, like blacks, face poverty, unemployment, undereducation, prejudice, and discrimination. Their life situations are stressful and complicate mental health problems. The President's Commission on Mental Health (1978) has noted the low quality and quantity of mental health services available to Hispanics, stating that Brandon

(1975), Kruger (1974), and Solis (1977) have found, given the few services to begin with, the rate of Hispanic utilization of these services is very low (about 50% of their representation in the population).

OTHER MINORITIES

Factors related to mental health and underutilization of mental health services among other racial minorities such as American Indians and Asian/Pacific-Americans are similar. The seriously inadequate conditions in which racial minorities live produce enormous stress. The effects of stress are compounded by the lack of understanding of cultural issues by service providers and by the lack of services to meet minorities' special needs.

THE ELDERLY

Abundant evidence proves that the elderly are one of the most underserved special population groups. Cohen (1977), for example, found that only 4% of the patients at outpatient mental health facilities were elderly. Butler and Lewis (1977) showed that among those seen in private psychiatric care, only about 2% were elderly. The low rate of utilization of mental health services by the elderly is not caused by an absence of mental health problems. Mental illness is in fact *more* prevalent among the elderly than among younger adults (e.g., Butler, 1975; Cohen, 1977; President's Commission on Mental Health, 1978). Cohen estimates about 15% to 25% of all elderly persons experience significant mental health problems. Persons over 65 years of age commit 25% of all suicides. Since the U.S. Census Bureau has projected that the elderly population is expected to more than double in the next few decades, their underutilization of services and high level of mental disorders present special problems. Expensive custodial institutions such as "nursing homes" and state hospitals have been overutilized as a substitute for appropriate medical intervention and community support. This practice is both inhumane and economically wasteful. Lives of dependency are substituted for lives of dignity. The "illderly" and "wellderly" tend to be lumped together, segregated from society, and mistreated. The fact that the most common emotional disorder of old age is curable depression remains ignored because dementias are all too often inappropriately assumed to be present. The "pseudodementias" crowd institutions, unnecessarily producing the shipwrecks of late life.

WOMEN

Unlike racial minorities and elderly populations, women, who represent over half the population of the United States (51.3%), are not a minority. In many areas of life—income, employment, legal rights—women are nevertheless in a disadvantaged position, which contributes to lowered self-esteem (Seidler-Feller, 1976), psychological disorders (Maracek, 1976), and mental illness (Davidson, 1977).

Mental health problems of women have been widely studied (e.g., Guttentag, Salasin, Legge, & Bray, 1976; President's Commission on Mental Health, 1978; Radloff, 1975; Weissman, 1975). Weissman, for example, found that 75% more women than men are admitted to hospitals for the treatment of depression. More than twice as many women as men are treated for depression in outpatient facilities. The President's Commission on Mental Health reported statistics from the National Institute of Drug Abuse stating that twice as many women as men use Valium and Librium (popular tranquilizers).

Spurlock (1977) reported that the mental health service delivery system for women is highly inadequate and marked by the same biases that help put women in a disadvantaged position in the first place. Most doctoral-level mental health professionals are male, and most patients are women. In the mental health work force, women are often segregated and stratified into low-status occupations. Mental health training programs have not made use of much of the new reserach of the past decade that relates to women (Benedek, 1977). The President's Commission on Mental Health (1978) reports that the American Psychological Association has documented sex biases in the therapeutic process among psychologists. This situation reinforces the powerlessness and alienation among women patients and may complicate recovery processes. Some therapists tend to be inattentive and disbelieving of external sources of anguish and anxiety faced by women. Adjustment to traditional roles by women may be stressed, while anger may be viewed as inappropriate and a sign of pathology. Male therapists who have not worked through these issues may inflict both countertransference distortions and cultural anthropocentricity on vulnerable women patients. Some problems are even more blatant. Women's claims of unrest and/or rape are often disbelieved. Sexual exploitation of women patients is also a serious problem. It is alleged that as many as 10% of male psychiatrists and psychologists have had sexual contact with women who have been in treatment with them (Kardiner et al., 1973; Halroyd & Brodsky, 1977). Whether the actual figure is lower is an irrelevancy. One case is one too many.

Thus, the mental health service delivery system either under-serves, is underutilized by, or is inappropriately designed to meet the needs of special population groups. For the working class and racial minorities, the underutilization of services may be due to the lack of understanding of class and cultural differences by mental health professionals. For the elderly and women, the primary problem is the inappropriateness of current services.

ASSUMPTION 3

In neighborhoods and communities throughout the U.S., a vast array of informal or lay community support systems exists. These systems include the help provided by friends, neighbors, clergy, natural helpers, mutual aid/self-help groups, ethnic, fraternal and social organizations, co-workers, etc. Despite abundant evidence of the importance of these support systems to individuals in need, community support systems are often ignored and/or bypassed by the formal bureaucratic mental health delivery system.

Community support systems provide important sources of mental health assistance. The term *community support systems* refers to such examples as:

- The woman in her 60s on the block to whom neighbors turn for help and support when their welfare checks are late.
- The clergyman to whom parishioners talk about their marital problems, worries about their children, or their sense of guilt and loss of meaning and belief.
- The widowed person's group that a church sponsors to provide mutual support and socialization.
- The neighbor who takes in the 14-year-old girl who has been thrown out of her house by her family.
- The pharmacist to whom customers talk about imagined somatic complaints and fears.
- The community organization that helps residents to develop a needed telephone crisis hotline.
- The ethnic organization that helps the middle-aged parent with the strains caused by value conflicts with their children.
- The co-worker who helps with the problems of caring for aged parents.

- The union shop steward who identifies channels for getting help for inattentiveness, or alcohol abuse that could produce job loss.

Kin, friends, neighbors, co-workers, clergy, sociocultural organizations, and mutual aid groups—all of which can provide meaningful support in times of need—are encompassed in community support systems. These support systems are "natural" in that the person-to-person caregiving efforts usually develop without professional support or assistance. Most organizational forms of community support systems, such as mutual aid groups and neighborhood organizations, similarly develop without professional intervention. Some forms of these support systems may develop in response to a specific societal problem—for example, the problem of divorce leading to support groups for the divorced—or in response to the lack of professional services to address a particular problem, such as a self-help group for bereaved parents.

Community support systems serve all of us to some degree, and in differing ways. More specifically, however, community support systems serve many population groups that are unable or frightened to secure professional help, or for whom professional services are lacking. Included among these are many ethnic and racial minority group members and elderly persons.

Community support systems can serve a preventive function by contributing to an individual's sense of well-being and of competent functioning. They can assist in reducing the negative consequence of stressful life events. Community support systems can offer help in a manner that is culturally acceptable. They can guide persons to needed professional help in a way that sustains pride and reduces stigma. The individuals seeking help can receive some level of support without being labeled "crazy" by anybody. Moreover, when professional aid is needed, the community can sanction such aid so there is no sense of being "weak" or "crazy." Diagnosis can be detoxified of stigma and brought closer to other medical issues if it is required. Finally, community support systems can be especially important for the chronically mentally ill, who need assistance in recovering from the isolation of institutional life.

The pertinence of community support systems to mental health is evident in the following statement in the recent report of the President's Commission on Mental Health:

> To be connected to others, to belong, to receive social support when it is needed and to be able to give it in return is an important part of mental health. What is more significant is that utilization of social and community support systems can provide for constructive innovations and systematic

change in the mental health system, moving toward a comprehensive
human service system with a holistic orientation that would remedy some
of the defects of our present fragmented and uncoordinated efforts. (President's Commission on Mental Health, 1978, p. 144)

Abundant research literature also documents the importance of community support systems (e.g., Breton, 1964; Caplan, 1974; Collins & Pancoast, 1976; Gartner & Reissman, 1977; Glazer, 1971; Hamburg & Killilea, 1979; Litwak, 1961; McKinlay, 1973; Mitchell, 1969; Pancoast, 1978; Silverman, 1978; Slater, 1970; Warren, 1977). During the 1960s, the work of Litwak, Mitchell, and others focused mainly on studying the patterns and nature of "networks of relationships." The seminal work of Caplan (1974) extended the concept of support systems to the mental health field. Rachelle Warren (1977) has argued that the strengthening of support systems can help individuals: (1) to gain a sense of control over their lives; (2) to reduce alienation from society; (3) to gain a capacity to solve new problems; and (4) to maintain the motivation to overcome the handicaps and frustrations of modern society. There is no way that one-to-one, doctor–patient relationships can substitute for these functions. There aren't enough doctors, and medicalization of social support helps in neither system. The time has come to cease perception of social support as competitive with medical psychiatric care. Neither can substitute for the other. Both are needed in their proper context.

Recent literature has emphasized specific roles and functions of support systems. Hamburg and Killilea (1979) reported that support systems modify the deleterious effects of life stress. A support system is especially effective as a buffer in times of crisis, enabling people to cope and adapt to change (e.g., Caplan & Killilea, 1976; Cassel, 1974; Warren & Waren, 1977).

Community support systems provide vital bridges among the individual, the environment, and service professionals. Collins and Pancoast (1976) argued that a community-based network of informal caregivers or "natural helpers" has a tremendous potential for delivery of mental health and other human services. Lee (1969) traced the important role of social networks in finding and selecting doctors who terminate pregnancies. Traunstein and Killilea (as discussed in Caplan & Killilea, 1976) describe how people in an upper-New York State community received service from their peers that paralleled and complemented the professional service network. Naparstek, Biegel, and Spence (1979) documented the important helping services being provided in urban ethnic communities by such informal sources as clergy, neighborhood leaders, and natural helpers, and the paucity of linkages between these informal networks and mental health professionals. Sarason, (1977) discussed the importance of kinship networks in the lives of the increasing number of single, widowed, or divorced individuals in our society. Some of these individuals will sustain acute depressions or other severe neuroses that call for professional help. Thus, both informal and formal support systems are critically important.

The nature and operation of community support systems will be further delineated through examination of three support system components: clergy, mutual aid/self-help groups, and natural helpers.

CLERGY

The border between religion and psychiatry has not always been a friendly place. Today's strain is trivial compared to the problems of the past. Less than five centuries ago schizophrenics and persons with hysterical and dissociative neuroses were being burnt at the stake as witches. From time to time their potential physicians were required to join them as heretics! Even today, clergymen may suspect that mental health professionals foster moral decay, and mental health professionals may regard the clergy as too welded to concepts of guilt, sin, and the supremacy of superego to be helpful in a treatment context. Yet this boundary that divides also connects. Psychiatrists have been described as "physicians to the soul." Clergymen are the key professionals in many neighborhoods.

Various scholars have written on the helping role of clergy in community mental health (e.g., Caplan, 1974; Clinebell, 1970; Cumming & Harrington, 1963; Haugk, 1976; Larson, 1968; Pargament, 1982; President's Commission on Mental Health, 1978; Veroff, Douvan, & Kulka, 1976). The importance of religious resources was recognized by the Joint Commission on Mental Illness and Health (1961), particularly in its final report, *Action for Mental Health,* in which it was stated that mentally troubled Americans turned most frequently to clergymen for help. Richard McCann (1962), in one of a series of studies undertaken for the Commission, examined the role of clergy in the use of mental health services. McCann found, through interviews with 160 individuals from a northeastern and a midwestern city, that although the majority of the respondents indicated a certain degree of independence in coping with their problems, they were more likely to seek help from a clergyman than from a psychiatrist. While 20 years have brought change, clergy remain an important source of counsel and referral for many Americans.

Cumming and Harrington (1963) interviewed clergymen from 59 churches and found that most of them were involved in counseling and making referrals of clients to other agencies. They also found that the clergyman, along with the physician, is the first contact made outside of the kinship and friendship circle during the onset of mental health problems. Veroff et al. (1976) found more people (39.2%) who said that they would turn to clergy if they had a problem than to any other professional, although other studies suggest that family doctors are selected (Spiro, Crocetti, Siassi, Ward, & Hansen, 1975).

Religious personnel and institutions, by their very nature, seem to foster support and trust among individuals, families, and neighbors (Caplan, 1974). They are thus an important community resource, which is underestimated and underutilized by community mental health agencies. "Churches and temples collectively represent a sleeping giant, a huge potential of barely tapped resources for fostering positive mental health," according to Clinebell (1970, p. 46).

The number of clergy in the United States is impressive: In 1972, there were 393,826 ordained clergymen of all faiths in the United States, including 235,189 affiliated with congregations. There were 328,657 separate congregations with an inclusive membership of 115,442,829 (Jacquet, 1972). The President's Commission on Mental Health noted that clergy and lay religious leaders are in daily face-to-face contact with hundreds of thousands of persons who are experiencing periods of stress caused by illness, injury and accidents, death, separation or divorce, unemployment, and other forms of loss and grief (President's Commission on Mental Health, 1978). Kenneth Haugk, reviewing contributions of churches and clergy to community mental health, called local congregations "a therapeutic community" in which there are many opportunities for support and prevention to take place (Haugk, 1976). Haugk reported that Gurin and Hollingshead and Redlich found the psychiatric professions to be disproportionately preferred by those of higher education and income, while clergy were used about evenly by all income groups and by all educational groups. Spiro, Crocetti, Siassi, Ward, and Hansen (1975) found this finding invalid among blue-collar workers. Haugk specifies numerous assets of clergy as help-givers: They are geographically well located and distributed; they do not charge fees; they have personal relationships with many of their parishioners; they need not wait for people to come and talk with them—they are expected to call on people—and there is little stigma attached to talking with a clergyman about problems; and they are principal "gatekeepers" in the helping system, uniquely positioned to pave the way to a referral because of their closeness to individuals in need and their professional authority.

The relationship between clergy and mental health professionals needs redefinition. The Community Support Systems Task Force of the President's Commission on Mental Health (1978) recommended that mechanisms be developed to "link the personnel and buildings owned by religious groups and institutions to community mental health centers and other social service agencies" (Vol. 2, p. 196). Obstacles often hinder or block these necessary linkages. Smith and Hobbs (1966) observed that the separation of mental health services from other people/service organizations and agencies—such as the churches—has hindered the delivery of appropriate help to people in need.

Cumming and Harrington (1963) report tension between clergy and mental health professionals. Whereas clergymen tended to make referrals of clients to mental health agencies, they did not receive appropriate referrals from mental health professionals. Insufficient personal contact between agency professionals and clergy was cited for this tension. "Social workers and psychiatrists who know a clergyman personally are more likely to exempt him from the stigma of 'judgmental clergyman,' and to consider him 'professionalized' or 'sophisticated' and thus to cooperate with him in the management of some clients" (Cumming & Harrington, 1963, p. 242). This tension between clergy and mental health professionals has been aggravated by competition for "motivated clients." Clergy seemed to experience less tension in dealing with lawyers, doctors, and other professionals when there was no question of overlapping expertise. Clergy experienced role conflict, according to the authors, vis-à-vis their role as referrer rather than direct helper. They seemed unsure which clients to refer, which clients not to refer, and how to refer without jeopardizing their role as a counselor. Their tension with human service professionals no doubt complicated this role conflict.

Larson (1968) reported significant disagreements between mental health professionals and clergy in their perception of each other's roles. In a study in which he sent psychiatrists and clergy six vignettes of persons experiencing varying degrees of emotional disturbance, Larson asked each respondent to assess the degree of mental illness, to specify the extent to which the respondent would become part of the therapeutic process, and to indicate to whom referrals ought to be made. In every instance, the psychiatrists were more likely to see the role of the clergy as referral agents only and to disagree significantly with the clergy's perception of their own role. In over 90% of the cases, psychiatrists were more likely to recommend psychiatric referral.

Perhaps ongoing dialogue can clarify mutual expectations. As the clergyman's role clarifies, increasing training, skill, and expertise in that role may increase the confidence of mental health professionals in their work with clergy.

MUTUAL AID/SELF-HELP GROUPS

Abundant literature exists to document the importance of self-help groups in community mental health (e.g., Caplan, 1974; Caplan & Killilea, 1976; Gartner & Reissman, 1977; Gussow & Tracy, 1978; President's Commission on Mental Health, 1978; Reissman, 1965; Silverman, 1970). One of the most intriguing aspects of the self-help group is that it is a dynamic process: A recipient of help can change roles and become a helper (Reissman, 1965). As members of a self-help group aid one another, they acquire positive reinforcement, either by identification with a fellow sufferer or by becoming "veterans" of the experience. Self-help groups are also significant because their affective and cognitive support is oriented towards shared goals, problems, or situations (Silverman, 1970). Self-help groups have been found to be particularly helpful in managing life cycle transitions, controlling deprivations and noxious habits, and changing lifestyles (Caplan & Killilea, 1976).

The danger of self-help groups is that persons who require professional help may be delayed from receiving adequate diagnosis and treatment. Some self-help groups can develop an arrogance and hostility to skilled professional help, which proves antitherapeutic. Proper linkages and understanding of how to make needed early referrals in a positive way are essential.

The President's Commission on Mental Health estimated that there may be more than a half million self-help groups in the United States today. These groups, according to Spiegel (1982), range from total institutions, such as Synanon, to subculture organizations such as Alcoholics Anonymous, to supplementary communities, such as Parents Without Partners, to life-transitions communities, such as ex-patient organizations. Self-help groups are important community resources that reach individuals who might not ordinarily go to a professional for help. Evidence also suggests that self-help groups can play a significant role in rehabilitating former mental patients, for whom inadequate aftercare has been well documented (President's Commission on Mental Health, 1978). Here, too, cooperative ties to the professional helping institutions are badly needed so that two-way referral can occur. Among the reasons for the effectiveness of self-help groups, according to Spiegel (1982), are: commonality of experience, mutual support, receiving help through giving it, collective willpower, information sharing, and goal-directed problem solving.

NATURAL HELPERS

Natural helpers exist at every socioeconomic level and in every community. Their role does not rely on education, age, sex, or social class. Natural helpers are "ordinary people" who are seen by others to be especially resourceful and empathetic (Pancoast, 1978). They are self-taught experts in their own field. They constantly seek to increase their usefulness and to improve their skills. Their interest and investment in those whom they help may be extremely high, just as with motivated professionals (Collins, 1973). Differences are in skill and knowledge, not in motivation and caring. Natural helping networks have central figures who, in addition to sharing their personal resources, also serve as linchpins, linking individual members of their networks who could mutually profit from exchanges (Pancoast, 1978).

There are a number of natural helping networks in any neighborhood. These networks tend to be of long duration and serve many purposes. Because of their idiosyncratic nature, they are sensitive to geographical, class, and ethnic differences. At their best they can react quickly to the changing needs of their network members (Collins & Pancoast, 1977).

Even so, natural networks should not be unduly romanticized. Some have also proven to be rigid, harshly judgmental, and insistent upon conformity. We commend their potential but with full awareness of their variety and possible negative features.

Natural helping networks exist in all types of settings. Natural helpers have been found in the tavern culture of homeless men and among severely disabled older adults living in single-room occupancy (SRO) hotels (Collins & Pancoast, 1976).

Experience indicates that professionals ought not to tamper or interfere with natural helping systems, but rather should develop selective linkages with positive systems where they exist (Naparstek & Biegel, 1979; Pancoast, 1978; Smith & Collins, 1979; Warren & Clifford, 1975). Numerous advantages accrue from such linkages. First, natural helpers can often reach individuals who would otherwise remain isolated and adrift. Second, forming partnerships with natural helpers can relieve problems of stigmatizing recipients of aid or creating dependencies upon formal services. Third, such linkages can provide information about formal services to a population that may not be using them because they do not know about them. Fourth, linkages can extend the service capacity of formal agencies (Pancoast, 1978). The President's Commission on Mental Health (1978) reports, however, that linkages between natural and professional helping networks are the exception rather than the rule. We have found that the vagueness about these networks, the tendency to idealize and romanticize, leave many professionals reluctant to develop such linkages.

Community support systems encompass many potential resources that could be useful in the delivery of mental health services. Yet these resources have not been effectively involved by mental health systems planners. Exhortatory rhetoric has tended to replace concrete program ties. The Report to the President from the President's Commission on Mental Health stated:

> In spite of the recognized importance of community supports, even those that work well are too often ignored by human service agencies. Moreover, many professionals are not aware of, or comfortable with, certain elements of community support systems. (1978, p. 15)

At least part of the problem is the government's policy of rewarding professionals for patient-contact hours and its failure to plan reimbursement mechanisms for time spent on links with informal helpers.

The Commission, as its first recommendation, proposed that:

> A major effort be developed in the area of personal and community supports which will: (a) recognize and strengthen the natural networks to which people belong and on which they depend; (b) identify the potential social support that formal institutions within communities can provide; (c) improve the linkages between community support networks and formal mental health services; and (d) initiate research to increase our knowledge of informal and formal community support systems and networks. (1978, p. 15)

We would strongly agree with the need for research to identify more concrete, specific natural helping systems that are effective, and the development of fiscal mechanisms to foster ties. Federal and state government pronouncements, marked by vague idealization and accompanied by fiscal disincentives, may retard research even more than disinterest on the part of concerned professionals. In this book, we will describe specific efforts to involve specific natural helper groups. Specificity and funding adequacy are the core issues.

Assumption 3 speaks to neighborhood systems that can be linked to mental health professional resources. The essentials are: specificity in identifying such resources; awareness of both liabilities and assets within each of the systems; realistic assessment of positive qualities, as well as limitations; and practical fiscal arrangements. All of these are necessities if the possiblities inherent in this assumption are to move beyond rhetoric.

ASSUMPTION 4

A sense of competency, self-esteem, and power is important to positive mental health within a community. Systems should be designed to build competency and to develop power for neighborhoods. This necessitates a radical change in the mutual roles of the community and professional institutions within the community mental health delivery system. The structures needed to develop an excellent psychiatric hospital differ from structures needed to develop links to a community.

The term competence may be interpreted differently in different social settings. In a technological society, competence might be considered synonymous with expertise in a particular field. In a society oriented towards moral concerns, competence may connote superior morals. For example, a judge might be expert in the law, but might be considered incompetent because of his moral weaknesses. Yet another meaning of competence would imply mastery of specific skills such as music, dance, athletics, and so forth.

In the mental health field, however, competence refers to an individual's ability to cope with day-to-day life events successfully. On a larger scale, focusing on the level of community, competence refers to the ability of a community to meet its needs and resolve its problems. In other words, competence means that a community has a sense of control over its environment. Such competence implies low levels of alienation. Confusion between competence required to render care to the severely ill (technologic competence) and competence to develop a meaningful community has led to rivalry where none need exist. Hospitals cannot build communities. Communities cannot operate hospitals. Both lack the respective specific competencies. The community mental health center at its worst offered incompetency in both spheres. Rarely has one institution simultaneously produced medical technologic competency and neighborhood-building competency.

Bloom (1977) believes that much of human misery is based on a lack of competence, including the lack of control over one's life, lack of effective coping strategies, and inherently low self-esteem. More and more professionals, he indicates, regard the building of individual and community competence as the major community mental health task of the immediate future. Bloom's analysis of a substantial body of research suggests that competence building can play a crucial role in dealing with the individual and social issues being faced in most communities.

Here is where professionals concerned solely with severe illness often split with professionals seeking to mitigate the discomfort of the "worried well" as well as to foster humane care for the chronically ill. There is no current evidence that the base rate of acute schizophrenia or of manic depressive disease (the two major functional psychoses) is altered by one's sense of competence. In so far as we now know, community building will not stamp out any of the known major psychiatric disorders. It may not even reduce incidence of any of these disorders. However, a competence-building, socially integrated neighborhood committed to caring for its members, and linked to psychiatric treatment programs, can foster rehabilitation and community care of the chronically ill. (See Spiro, 1980b, for a fuller analysis of the false hopes and real prospects in prevention programs.)

Ryan (1971), discussing the relationship between competency and power, finds that the degree to which a person is powerful is proportional to the degree to which he is more likely to be "mentally healthy"; to the degree that he is powerless, he is likely to be lacking "mental health." Ryan feels mental health services should be oriented to increasing community power through community organizations and through the fostering of political, lobbying, and publication activities by mental health professionals. (We would note that Ryan's "lack of mental health" is quite different from the presence of severe mental illness.)

The 1972 *Report of the American Psychiatric Association Task Force to Develop a Position Statement on Community Mental Health Centers* states that:

> The affluent and the sophisticated significantly control their health and mental health resources. This has not been true for poor people and many middle class people. It is widely believed that control of one's circumstances and of one's community enhances the sense of identity of a group, its cohesion, competency, and mental health. This striving for control can have useful effects on the development of community mental health centers and on other health programs by contributing to the ordering of priorities that are meaningful to and supportable by the consumer of services. Community development and community organization that lead to community control are often justified as preventive efforts in mental health. (pp. 10–11)

How is such community power to be achieved? To overcome the problem of powerlessness and alienation of individuals and communities, citizen participation and community action programs were deemed essential in the 1960s, a period during which there was a tremendous increase in such programs. Citizen participation in such public programs was an important variable of their success. But as Spiegel (1968) noted, the demand on all sectors of government for action mitigated against the time-consuming process of genuine citizen participation. The federal government purported to support the desirability of social planning and participation, but made it impossible to achieve because of bureaucratic red tape and unrealistic deadlines.

A "top-down" approach proved unworkable because the government failed to provide mechanisms to devolve power to citizens at the neighborhood level. Although beginning attempts were made to involve citizens, rigid guidelines from Washington prevented needed adaptation of "bottom-up" strategies. In the end, the federal mandates and control made genuine citizen participation unworkable. In addition, federal targeting of poor and minority neighborhoods, to the exclusion of the working classes, added unnecessarily to feelings of alienation in those communities and damaged the formation of a majority consensus, which was needed for the continuation of the programs.

Government mandates often attempted to devolve power to areas where community competence is an irrelevancy. The HSAs had persons making crucial technical decisions about complex hospital management guided by "professional planners" whose expertise was no greater than the citizen groups they advised. Ignorance was often equaled only by arrogance as hospital costs spiraled upward. In the meantime, those same citizens had vitually no input into that area in which their competence was very high: the development of their own neighborhoods. Expressways, zoning changes, urban renewal—or destruction—projects were dropped like cluster bombs by government bureaucrats, while citizens were left with "responsibility" to decide where radio-isotope labs would be permitted and how to treat psychiatric inpatients.

Only Franz Kafka could supply the appropriate prose to describe the insanity of these 1970s efforts. People were allowed to play doctor-for-a-day and decide the efficacy of and need for cardiac surgery, but they were denied a voice in whether their neighborhood should be demolished to make room for glass-plated, anonymous high-rise apartments! Presumably they lacked "competence" to join in decision making that affected their daily lives. Both roles contributed to a sense of alienation and incompetence.

How ironic that mental health professionals, often deprived of authority to manage their own hospitals, have been given sanction to make some rather basic community decisions in many areas. Perhaps the madness is best described as "reciprocal incompetence."

   To meet the "health" as opposed to the "illness" needs of the community adequately, residents must achieve empowerment—that is, a sense of equity, security, and sufficiency (see chapter 2). Empowerment need not be acquired at the expense of agencies and institutions. In fact, agencies can benefit from community empowerment. Agencies often have difficulty attracting a sufficient number of clients in urban communities, where the values of pride and privacy make people unwilling and unable to seek help unless the worsening of their problem forces them to do so. We favor the same principles of autonomy and devolution of self-determining power to institutions as to neighborhoods. In a pluralistic society, self-determining agencies and institutions may compete in the survival of the fittest as they seek to link to empowered neighborhoods. Government is equally incompetent in management and decision making for both groups!

   A community-directed empowerment approach is thus vital for dealing with issues of prevention and for enhancing community strengths. To examine appropriate community and professional roles, it may be helpful to review two conceptions of social welfare that seem to dominate professional thinking in the United States today: the "residual" and the "institutional." Wilensky and Lebeaux feel that the first approach

> holds that social welfare institutions should come into play only when the normal structures of supply, the family, and the market, break down. The second ["institutional" conception], in contrast, sees the welfare service as the normal "first line" function of modern industrial society. (1965, p. 138)

   These concepts are regarded as a compromise between the values of economic individualism and free enterprise on the one hand, and security, equality, and humanitarianism on the other. Current social work practice has tried to combine the two, but with further industrialization, the second is likely to prevail.

   Although few today would doubt the necessity and responsibility of the government to provide social services to those who need them, there has been too much emphasis on the decline of the family, church, and neighborhood, and the presumed inability of these institutions to survive. Believing these entities to be unimportant, the designers of public programs tend to weaken and undermine them, thus creating a self-fulfilling prophecy. There is a certain self-interest identifiable when government bureaucracies reach such conclusions. Neighborhoods are incompetent (so we are told), institutions and agencies need tight (government) reins (so we are told)—*voila!* Only a bigger government bureaucracy can manage all! We question both the conclusions and the self-serving—though perhaps unconscious—motives that may lead to those conclusions.

Rapid changes in modern American society, and the problems inherent in these changes, require strong families, churches, and neighborhoods. While recognizing the permanence and the importance of professional social services, we believe that they should be designed to strengthen and empower families, churches, and neighborhoods as first-line help-providers. Services today fail to operate in this manner. The importance of neighborhood and neighborhood-based networks is not recognized. Agencies often deliver services without a clear sense of mission, goals, and relationship to the community. There is widespread lack of understanding about how to achieve the objective of neighborhood empowerment.

Neighborhood empowerment requires a radical change from the goal of mere community "participation" in services. Roland Warren believes the mental health movement has had strong citizen participation from its inception; however, participation has been guided more by the legitimacy and support functions of prominent citizens who could be recruited to endorse mental health legislation programs than by any sense of direct accountability to a service clientele.

Practical difficulty arises in distinguishing between a community decision and a professional decision. Sarason offers some advice:

> Whenever there is a gross discrepancy between community needs and available services, it is a matter of community policy, not professional policy, how the available service should be distributed and what alternative steps should be taken to meet community needs. (Sarason, 1977, p. 217)

Professional decision making belongs in professional institutions. Community decision making is needed for community policy.

CONCLUSION

It is evident that our present mental health system is inadequate to meet the mental health needs of its people. In our view, mental health services should:

1. Understand and account for the pluralistic nature of American society.
2. Be designed to account for ethnic, class, racial, sex, and age differences in the population.
3. Build upon the strengths and helping resources in the community.

4. Develop linkages between the professional mental health delivery system and the informal service network.
5. Increase the community's sense of competence and power.
6. Allow control by the community for neighborhood programs and services, and allow control by professionals for high-technology institutions.
7. Be integrated with the human services system.

A model based on these objectives is presented in the following chapter.

CHAPTER 7

The Model
A Community Mental Health Empowerment Model

INTRODUCTION

The Community Mental Health Empowerment Model, which will be described in this chapter, emphasizes the unique strengths of city neighborhoods so that neighborhood support systems are mobilized and networks are created to link professional and informal service systems. The objective is to identify and overcome obstacles that prevent community residents from seeking and receiving help. This model differs from other community mental health approaches in that it is a capacity-building process for neighborhoods and it is directed by a local community organization, which then is linked to health resources. Through this process, neighborhood residents become aware of their abilities to shape services to meet community needs. This can lead to rational redirection of existing services and creation of new programs to meet newly identified needs.

Even though the community mental health movement has been a vast improvement over prior public mental health efforts in communities, it has failed to base programs on the specific strengths, resources, and diversities of unique local communities. A neighborhood contains the "locality-relevant" institutions that connect the individual to the fabric of society: church, school, community and civic associations, pharmacist, physician, small businesses and more. Less visibly, neighborhoods contain informal helping networks that aid individuals in coping with the problems and crises of daily life.

City neighborhoods have been cast in a pejorative light recently, with attention focused almost exclusively on ugly problems such as crime, unemployment, and physical blight—problems to be solved by outside government institutions. In the designing of mental health and human service programs, the strengths of neighborhoods have often been overlooked. It is on neighborhood strengths—and their potential for enhancement—that this model has been constructed. This frees health resources for doing what they do best: practicing high-quality medicine rather than pretending to be "community programs."

Despite abundant evidence of the importance of neighborhood attachment and neighborhood-based informal support systems, "community" mental health programs have often been "parachuted" into localities without adequate consultations with residents and with few, if any, linkages to informal community support systems. Boundary lines of community mental health catchment areas have even been drawn so that they cut across established neighborhoods irrationally. The positive identification of community residents with their neighborhoods has not been employed to overcome personal and institutional obstacles to seeking and receiving help.

The 1975 amendments to the Community Mental Health Act required that federally funded community mental health centers develop governing boards with a majority of members selected from among nonservice providers; in other words, community residents. In reality, center directors have often selected well-known community personalities who are unlikely to "make waves" in their operations. Responsibility for community contact and involvement has been compartmentalized in one individual or in one office. Community control of specialized health institutions proved a farce. It redirected neighborhood residents into playing "doctor-for-a-day" while ignoring their real expertise in their own neighborhood. We propose *real* community involvement that permeates all parts of a neighborhood unit, while specialty psychiatry is practiced in a linked, specialized resource. This makes possible a genuine partnership between the neighborhood unit and the community. Among the advantages of such involvement are that it:

- Helps overcome the negative attitudes that have been attached to getting help for mental illness in some communities.
- Increases utilization of services.
- Helps reach people earlier in their need.
- Provides a basis for programming in the areas of prevention and deinstitutionalization.
- Creates a political constituency for mental health.

The pluralistic approach to provision of mental health and social services in the United States has resulted, as might be expected, in a patchwork crazy quilt of public and private programs with varying patterns of accountability, funding, eligibility criteria, and service provision. Mental health services, for example, may be supplied to a single neighborhood by a combination of state, county, and city governments and/or private agencies. Funding may come from a dizzying array of sources, each with its own funding mechanisms. One community mental health center might receive money from: federal, state, and local governments; the United Way; national and local foundations; fees; grants; contracts; purchases of service; insurance reimbursements; and more. Regulations, eligibility criteria, funding levels, and funding periods also vary. This adds up to a whole array of legal, fiscal, and administrative barriers to seeking and receiving help. In addition, opportunities for waste or misapplication of funds are burgeoning. So far, the principal effort to rationalize this confusion has been the "case management" approach. This approach, at best, helps selected clients but does not attack the source of the predicament: the system. At worst, it just adds one more level to an already overly complex system.

The Community Mental Health Empowerment Model, instead of identifying an individual as the client for neighborhood efforts, addresses the *system* as the client. That is, the agencies, community residents, and helpers within a geographic area (the neighborhood) are identified as a collective client beset by administrative, fiscal, and legal obstacles that have hampered the effective functioning of community mental health programs. Conversely, identified, severely ill, acute patients are treated as medically ill patients in high-technology medical resources. They are not bounced around social agencies as "clients." Once labeling becomes necessary, diagnosis should be done by experts who follow up with effective treatment. The appropriate use of appropriate modalities for appropriate individuals is a key feature of the model.

The model recognizes the necessity of addressing the system's obstacles, all of which have macrocomponents external to the neighborhood. Since no single sector—public, private, or community—possesses sufficient resources to solve the complex web of issues confronting community mental health, we advocate the establishment of partnerships among all sectors, including new intergovernmental partnerships, and emphasis on private institutions and agencies.

The model is, in other words, a systems approach. The neighborhood is conceived of as the key element on which helping networks are based and from which helping networks flow. The neighborhood will be seen to function in five ways:

1. As a locus for community-focused services.
2. As a support system and vehicle for the development of professional and lay helping networks.
3. As the basis for the development of neighborhood-relevant
   mental health programming.
4. As a means for citizen/patient involvement.
5. As the basis for empowerment of citizens in mental health.

One must not focus on preconceived specific issues in particular
population groups in preference to neighborhood process issues. We
believe that neighborhood people must have the opportunity to bring to
the surface the issues relevant to them. Mental health institutions and
agencies often distort their image of a community through the lens of
their own predetermined institutional needs, an "institutional imperative." Agency personnel and government civil servants, who usually
serve more than one neighborhood, cannot be expected to possess the
unique vision required to comprehend a community's perception of its
own needs; nor can they authentically represent a community. There is
a "blender" process that homogenizes neighborhoods and loses individual neighbhorhood priorities in favor of institutional priorities. We
will discuss how our demonstration project impacted on the specific
mental health issues that residents identified as their local priorities
rather than focusing on preselected issues in specific groups.

This model, it will be recalled, was developed through work
recently completed on a four-year research and demonstration grant
provided by the National Institute of Mental Health. The two urban
ethnic neighborhoods, South East Baltimore and the Southside of Milwaukee, are both stable, working-class areas with high concentrations
of white ethnic populations. The Milwaukee community is predominantly Polish; the Baltimore area contains Polish, German, Italian,
Ukranian, Greek, and Lithuanian populations. More detailed descriptions of the two communities and the programs developed there are
offered in chapters 9, 10, and 11.

Although the model was orginally developed for use in urban ethnic neighborhoods, we believe that the process described may be readily adapted to other types of communities. Discussion of key issues in
using the model, as well as limitations, follows in chapter 12.

The neighborhood is the locus of operations for both the community-focused professional and lay helping networks. In Figure 1 we
have identified a lay and a professional helping network. The lay network includes those helpers who provide support services on a voluntary basis to individuals in the community. Lay helpers may have

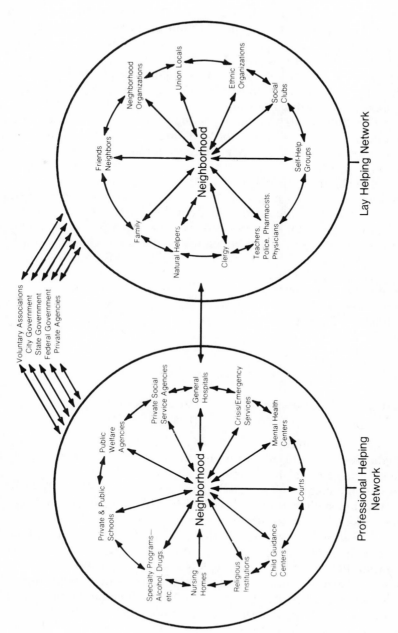

Figure 1. Neighborhood Mental Health Empowerment Model.

professional training, but the helping services they provide are an adjunct and not a principle part of their professional training and practice. For example, physicians may provide informal counseling for their patients. The professional network consists of those paid to provide support services to individuals in the community. These support services are provided in an agency or institutional context, usually by professionally trained persons.

The double arrows signify actual and potential communications channels and linkages between and among the various helpers, as well as to the macrosystem, which represents the larger forces that impact on relationships.

The Community Mental Health Empowerment Model is a process model, not a program model. As such, it cannot be replicated step-by-step. It must be developed over time through a series of stages. Thus, the description that follows is not intended as a recipe or a manual of "how-to's." It is a report of benchmarks in a process that was developed in our efforts to achieve certain goals. The intention is that the principles of the model should be applied to specific settings, with actual implementation strategies to be worked out to suit the needs of a particular area or situation. In presenting these strategies, we will first state objectives, then specify some possible implementation tactics.

OBJECTIVE

To Create Awareness by Neighborhood Residents of the Neighborhood Strengths and Needs

Organizationally, it is most logical for the initiating entity (which might be—to name just a few possibilities—a university, a hospital, a community mental health center, or a social agency) to work through an existing community-based organization (as we did in Baltimore) or to develop such a group (as we did in Milwaukee). Depending on the particular community, the sponsoring organization might be a neighborhood improvement association, a church group, or an ethnic club. By placing sponsorship and ownership of the process squarely with the community from the beginning, it is asserted as an axiom that residents have the strength and resources to define their own needs and capacities for themselves. At the same time, since the model involves building partnerships, the sponsoring organization must be willing to collaborate with other organizations and to share credit and blame for successes and failures.

When the initiating group involves a medical college, as was the case in Milwaukee, it is particularly important to back out of the way early and leave authority with community process-oriented personnel. The stronger the initiating entity, the more important it is to avoid "overwhelming" the neighborhood with ideas and concepts. Neighborhood process is the key. Creation of clear boundaries between the medical institution and neighborhood entity makes it possible for medical officials to step out of the way and let linkages develop. Giving neighborhood process workers effective governing control over high technology medical resources (the 1960s process) is a certain way to subvert this process, confuse needed boundaries, and destroy meaningful partnership.

Self-assessment is an extremely important and difficult matter. If someone from a mayor's office says that people in "Neighborhood A" have emotional problems and need services, then that neighborhood tends to be labeled as a "problem area" with the attendant stigma. If, instead, people in a neighborhood talk with their leaders, doctors, pharmacists, school personnel, human service workers, and natural helpers, and find out for themselves that residents are experiencing a variety of problems, not only have they defined the neighborhood's condition for themselves, but they have also begun to take responsibility for dealing with that problem. This reinforces the strength of the community while paving the way for needed attention to community problems. Using a clinical analogy, we know that to help someone, we must begin with his or her presentation of the problem, not our own. But once the problem is presented, we don't ask the patient to engage in complex diagnostic procedures like cardiac catheterization or to perform heart surgery on themselves.

In this methodology, it is recognized that action research is an indispensable tool for self-assessment. It was decided to involve community residents, directed by a task force of residents, in the gathering of data on help-giving and help-receiving in the neighborhood. They did this by collecting "objective" statistical figures and by conducting "subjective" interviews with community leaders and helpers. Once the gathering and analyzing of materials was under way, issues were clarified and action plans were developed by the Task Force to address the needs that had been identified. Thus even the classic "entry" and "diagnosis" steps of community development entailed neighborhood involvement from the outset.

For success in the process, the community residents needed to develop linkages with professional mental health and human service systems. Involvement of a wide variety of service agencies was required. To achieve this, an inventory was made of all local human service agencies. A Professional Advisory Committee (PAC) was then formed to advise the Task Force. Professionals who held decision-making positions in their agencies or institutions were purposely selected for the PACs so that they would have the capacity later to help commit resources to needed projects. It was understood from the start that the PAC would function in an advisory capacity to the Task Force, not as a directive force. The PAC would meet only as needed. Individual PAC members would be further involved as Task Force committees were formed to develop action plans.

OBJECTIVE

TO STRENGTHEN THE NEIGHBORHOOD LAY HELPING NETWORK

The helping process usually begins with relatives, friends, and neighbors. Next, a person in need tends to turn to a community professional such as a clergyman, teacher, or family physician. These people are the "gatekeepers." Since the goal was to enable people to seek help more effectively and sooner, we began where the helping process begins: the informal neighborhood helping network. Despite an early assumption that the neighborhood helping network was a coherent system, neighborhood helpers were not really linked to one another. The helpers were uncovered in the pilot neighborhoods because residents identified them as helpers, not because they formed a coherent system. The helpers involved in aiding community residents did not usually know each other and did not usually work together. The objective was to strengthen the lay helping network and to help residents acquire confidence in their ability to deal with mental health issues as non-professionals so that they would be able to interact with mental health professionals as bonafide partners. We recognized the fragility of lay helping networks and the dangers of tampering insensitively with them. It was important for the lay helpers to work on their own until they felt professional consultation with PAC members was needed. The lay helping network was strengthened through involvement by informal helpers in various Task Force activities such as: needs assessment, planning and development of demonstration programs, implementation and evaluation of programs. A dividend was the creation of awareness by lay helpers of each other's abilities, contributions, and talents: the development of a true network.

The process, then, was for the Task Force, including the neighborhood's helpers and leaders, to collect data, analyze it, and set priorities for intervention by the community. Working committees were then set up to develop demonstration programs. Planning committees were initially composed of neighborhood helpers and leaders. At a mutually agreed upon point in the process, members of the PAC were brought in as advisors to the planning committee.

Development of each intervention program served as a "means" as well as an "end." The end was achieved because intervention programs—whether they were self-help groups, family communications seminars, or crisis hotlines—addressed a specific need that had been identified by the community Task Force in collaboration with the PAC. The means—namely, the planning and development process—achieved the end of enhancing the capacity of lay people, first to work together and then to work in concert with the professionals as full partners. Involvement and participation were the key words. Things were not done "to" the community. The neighborhood residents were the ultimate "initiators."

OBJECTIVE

To Strengthen the Professional Helping Network

Professionals in the Community Mental Health Empowerment Model are advisors. This is a deviation from the traditional model in which citizens serve as advisors to a mystifying technical professional process. In the formation of a PAC, we discovered that the fragmented and uncoordinated professional helping system was strengthened by bringing together professionals who worked in a common locality yet had rarely, if ever, been in regular contact with one another. Although PAC members did not initially attend community board meetings, community residents did attend—and chair—PAC meetings. The purpose was to enable the community to develop its confidence and expertise so that residents could eventually work in a parity relationship with professionals. Serendipitously, we found that the structure was professionally "seductive." Professionals heard about intriguing community activities through the PAC, and increased their involvement. At the same time, community lay helpers acquired more and more legitimacy in the professionals' eyes. Gradually, mutually agreeable means through which professionals could increase their support for the lay network were developed without the professionals overwhelming the residents or "taking over" control of meetings or operations.

OBJECTIVE

To Form Linkages between the Lay and Professional Helping Networks

First, Task Force program committees were formed, then Task Force members invited professionals to work with the committees. By then, the PAC meeting process had sensitized most of the professionals to the capacity of the community to develop effective programs. The two systems were ready to develop a partnership, fully aware of their differing roles and agendas.

The concept of cosponsorship of programs broadened the appeal of and added an aura of legitimacy to the interventions. A publicity brochure for an *Eating Together* program for the elderly would list all the churches, agencies, and groups that were supporting the project. A socialization center for former psychiatric hospital patients would be set up in a church and run by the community with professional consultation and assistance. The system thus decreased the stigma attached to seeking help, linked lay and professional services effectively, and extended the resources of community agencies. It also met the goals of community and agency support.

OBJECTIVE

To Link the Lay and Professional Helping Networks and the Macrosystem

Once the neighborhood empowerment process is on its way, the community needs to examine the larger forces that impact on the process and represent resources, obstacles, and incentives to the institutionalization of the empowerment process. Task Force and PAC members in our pilot communities gathered a data base of information on state and local mental health and human services plans, United Way funding patterns, agency program plans, and pending major legislation. Local sources of funding were scouted. Linkages were established with local foundations, industry, and other funding institutions and organizations. This stage of the process was critical and must be recognized as such if accomplishments in the process are to be rendered long-lasting. A word of warning: This project had the benefit of a Washington-based, initiating organization (the Washington Public Affairs Center of the University of Southern California) with a history of successful ties to the federal establishment. Other initiating entities may have to utilize ingenuity, hire or "borrow" professional expertise in "grantsmanship" to deal with the multiplicity of funding possibilities.

CONCLUSION

We have described a model characterized by involvement of community residents as prime movers in assessing neighborhood needs and establishing neighborhood helping networks. The duality of the system is particularly important. Neighborhood residents were not trying to create outpatient diagnostic centers, inpatient units, or medication follow-up programs. They operated in their field of expertise, their own neighborhoods. Physicians expert in acute psychiatric care operated in their field of expertise. "Docking mechanisms" brought these subsystems together. The fact that neither subsystem had the authority or expectation to control the other smoothed the way for meaningful "docking mechanisms." No one threatened anyone else. Community "green berets" were not going to take over decision making in medical practice. Doctors were not going to dictate neighborhood policy. Respect for boundaries permitted both the needed differentiation of services and the formation of nonthreatening linkages. The model contrasts with both the blurred boundaries that characterized the programs of the 1960s and the institutionally dictated approaches of the 1970s that largely ignored community and neighborhood.

The focus of the next chapter is on methodology and initial research findings, which will serve both to provide further elucidation of the genesis of the Empowerment Model and to provide a reference point for chapters 9 and 10 on the demonstration programs.

CHAPTER 8

First Stages

Methodology, Organization, and Evaluative Data Prior to Empowerment

OVERVIEW

The Neighborhood and Family Services Project began as a four-year National Institute of Mental Health grant awarded from 1976–1980 and initiated when the senior author of this volume was at the National Center for Urban Ethnic Affairs. Drs. Naparstek and Spiro developed the original project design. This was an action research and demonstration project intended to:

1. Reduce negative attitudes among ethnic working-class neighborhoods towards mental health issues and mobilize such neighborhoods around those issues.
2. Develop model programs and effective service delivery systems that overcome current obstacles and are more congruent with the lifestyle of ethnic working-class populations.
3. Develop policy initiatives on the local, state, and national levels to institutionalize project findings in support of neighborhood-based community mental health services.

The very first stage, the predemonstration first year of the project, was utilized to develop organizational structures established to collect data and to begin program planning. Dr. Biegel joined the project at this time as Project Director and was responsible for implementing and directing project activities throughout the entire four years. Development, implementation, and evaluation of demonstration projects followed in succeeding years.

The first step was to identify the neighborhoods that would serve as the loci for the project. We originally sought two demonstration neighborhoods meeting these basic criteria: (1) an urban setting; (2) a

101

significant percentage of residents of Southern-and/or Eastern-European background; (3) a strong sense of neighborhood identity; and (4) a viable community umbrella organization to be linked to the project.

South East Baltimore, Maryland, fulfilled all criteria and became the first locus. The second site, in Providence, Rhode Island, also met the criteria, but events that will be related later prevented locating there. After one of the authors moved to Milwaukee as Chairman of the Medical College of Wisconsin, Department of Psychiatry, it was decided to seek a locus in this city. Although the Southside neighborhood in Milwaukee lacked an umbrella group, it was otherwise ideal. Project staff, therefore, helped to organize the South Community Organization, Inc. (SCO). Medical College staff remained out of the way so that SCO could evolve as a free-standing organization. SCO is now well on its way to being an independent, ongoing community group. SCO and Baltimore's South East Community Organizations (SECO) directed each respective project and received funding on a subcontract basis to hire local staff and cover expenses. The professional costs were kept very low to develop models "exportable" to neighborhoods for whom no grant money is available. .

Professionals in each community served on a Professional Advisory Committee (PAC) for the community groups. Both the community and PAC groups reviewed data findings, set priorities as needs were identified, and determined mechanisms for addressing those needs. A series of demonstration projects were then designed by the communities with PAC consultants. Although identified problems and needs in each city were similar, priorities and strategies in each city differed.

EVALUATION AND DATA COLLECTION BEFORE THE INTERVENTION

Initial evaluation focused on the following:

1. What *strengths* and *problems* exist in these two ethnic neighborhoods? Who defines these strengths and problems?
2. What professional and lay community helping *networks* exist; how are they linked and how are these networks *utilized* by community residents to meet needs?
3. What *obstacles* prevent individuals from seeking and receiving help?
4. What role does *ethnicity* play in problem identification and the use of lay/professional helping networks?
5. What role does *community attachment/affiliation* play in problem identification and the use of lay/professional helping networks?

Evaluation Objectives

The first objective was an accurate assessment of the strengths, needs, and resources of the target communities. We conducted two sets of interviews: one with a random sample of residents, a second with people recognized as community helpers and leaders. Statistical data provided additional information and served as a check on the subjective opinions of interviewees.

The data collection was also designed to facilitate organizing efforts. Legitimacy and credibility were needed in both neighborhoods. Otherwise, the research could have alienated neighborhood residents. This would have produced resistance and certain failure during the action phases of the work. SECO and SCO were never rubber-stamp organizations for staff efforts. They held decision-making control within the boundaries of the grant. They consistently challenged staff assumptions and directed research and its applications in programs. SCO and SECO linked project staff and bonafide community leaders and helpers. As a result, SCO and SECO became the major vehicles for legitimacy in their respective neighborhoods.

Most important, one must never forget that initial data collection is part of an entry process. If the community is not involved at each step, the most precise objective data cannot compensate for the failed entry process.

As intended, the research served as a tool for planning and program development by community and PAC groups. Additional data was analyzed by staff. This report is separately available (Naparstek, Biegel, & Spence, 1979). Because the community evaluation is a useful "initiating" task that provides vital diagnostic information for later tasks, we present here a brief summary of that longer report. Several of these data collection methods are low-cost methods applicable without special federal funding.

Evaluation Methodolgy

Three principal data sources were utilized:

1. *Statistical Data.* Four types of statistical data were collected.
   a. *Census Data.* The NIMH Demographic Profile System, based on 1970 Census Data, contains 130 variables (demographic, socioeconomic, cultural, etc.) from published and upublished census data available on a census tract basis and compiled for each mental health catchment area in the United States. We rearranged this NIMH data so that we could examine both individual neighborhoods or subareas in each city, and then the entire target area.

Comparisons were then made by city, county, state, and U.S. bases. By looking at a single table we could thus examine the distribution of particular variables on the neighborhood, city, county, state, and U.S. levels. The data describe the target areas in terms of ethnicity, socioeconomic status, household composition and family structure, residential lifestyle, type of housing, community stability, and populations with high potential need for health, welfare, and related services in the community.

b. *Social Indicator Data.* These included: birth, death, and health statistics; Social Security and welfare recipients; juvenile and adult crime; and school attendance and disciplinary statistics.

In Baltimore, birth, death, and health statistics were drawn from publications of the Bureau of Biostatistics, Baltimore City Health Department. In Milwaukee, they were provided by the State of Wisconsin, Department of Health and Social Services.

Social Security statistics in both cities came from the Social Security Administration, Department of Health, Education and Welfare. Welfare statistics in both cities were provided by their respective Departments of Social Services. Juvenile crime statistics for Baltimore came from the Maryland Department of Juvenile Services. Adult crime statistics were provided by the Baltimore City Police Department. The Milwaukee Police Department provided crime statistics for all age groups. Respective public school systems in the two cities provided attendance and disciplinary data.

c. *Data on Utilization of Mental Health Services.* One of our major assumptions was that white ethnic working-class populations have underutilized traditional mental health services. To document this in Maryland, we obtained mental health admission and termination data on a census tract basis from the *Case Register* maintained at the Maryland Department of Health and Mental Hygiene. In Milwaukee, similar mental health data were obtained from the Milwaukee County Mental Health Complex data bank, developed at the Medical College of Wisconsin.

d. *Data on Ethnicity of Agency Clientele.* The data above told us where people go for help, but did not show clients' ethnic identities. We asked selected mental health and human service agencies to add some questions on ethnicity to their intake procedure for a specified temporary period, usually one to two months. This mechanism gave us some indication of the percentage of total intake that were of foreign stock or self-identified as ethnic.

2. *Community Resident Survey.* Random samples consisting of 198 adult (age 18 and older) community residents in Baltimore, and 194

adult community residents in Milwaukee were interviewed face-to-face using the Kish selection process. A pretested instrument taking approximately 1 hour to administer was used. Subcontracted professional research organizations conducted the interviews under the guidance of project research staff. The survey instrument focused upon personal problems the interviewees had experienced, where they went for help, their attitudes towards help-seeking and receiving, their opinions of the problems of other community residents, and aspects of neighborhood attachment and ethnicity.

3. *Community Leader and Helper Survey.* Over 250 community leaders and helpers in Baltimore and Milwaukee were interviewed. Interviewees included clergy, natural helpers, neighborhood leaders, pharmacists, physicians, human service agency staff, and school personnel. (See appendix for survey instrument.)

The survey instrument utilized approximately 100 open- and closed-ended, pretested questions, and took 1 hour to administer. It was administered to 100% sample of leaders and helpers within selected neighborhoods of the target area. Refusal rates averaged below 25%. The survey instrument focuses on problems and use of helping networks for teens, families, the separated and divorced, and the elderly.

The survey included emphasis upon the following areas:

a. Demographic, social, cultural, and economic characteristics of the helpers and leaders (hereafter identified as "helpers").
b. Helpers' roles in helping individuals with problems.
c. Roles the helpers' organizations (churches, neighborhood groups, agencies, etc.) play in the helping process.
d. Knowledge of the problems of teenagers, families, the separated and divorced, the elderly, and the widowed in the community.
e. Helpers' definitions of problems. Do different groups of helpers define problems differently?
f. Knowledge of lay and professional helping networks. How, when, and for what problems are those networks utilized? Which resources are felt to be most helpful?
g. Knowledge of obstacles that prevent utilization of helping networks.
h. Specification of three major community issues.

INITIAL FINDINGS: THE "PRE" STUDIES

The Community Leader and Helper Survey was analyzed extensively and served as the basis for intervention strategies during the demonstration phase of the project. The focus of this brief presentation of research findings will be on that survey. A complete report of the findings has been presented elsewhere (Naparstek, Biegel, & Spence, 1979). Specific definitions and research criteria are available in these documents and will not be repeated here.

THE SEVEN INTERVIEW GROUPS (CLERGY, HUMAN SERVICE AGENCY PROFESSIONALS, NATURAL HELPERS, NEIGHBORHOOD LEADERS, PHARMACISTS, PHYSICIANS, AND SCHOOL PERSONNEL)

In both Baltimore and Milwaukee, the natural helpers tend to be women and the neighborhood leaders tend to be men. Natural helpers, following sex role norms, tend to help individuals with their personal problems, while the neighborhood leaders are more involved with broad community issues. People tend to come to natural helpers for personal assistance. Fewer neighborhood leaders say that people seek them out for help. Natural helpers generally know more about individual problems and the resources available to address them than neighborhood leaders do. On the other hand, neighborhood leaders have more extensive knowledge of community issues and are more knowledgeable about individuals involved with those issues. They have the, least knowledge of all interview groups about the problems of families and of the separated and divorced. Neighborhood leaders do know about the problems of teenagers, possibly because teen problems often become a community issue. Neighborhood leaders most frequently stated that there are insufficient services to address teenagers' problems.

The role of the natural helpers seems to be an extension into the community of women's caretaker role in the private domain of the family. The neighborhood leaders' functioning reflects the traditional norm, which sees men handling the affairs of the public domain. One result of this sex role division is that natural helpers, particularly in Baltimore, appear to be much more sensitive to individuals and to the impact of neighborhood issues on individuals. In the Baltimore target area, which has been experiencing significant change and where there are more severe problems than in the Milwaukee target area, natural helpers were the only ones who rated the neighborhood poorly, specifying that changes have created a poorer environment. The natural helpers in Baltimore were the sole group expressing substantial doubt about whether or not people with problems seek help. They also observed that their neighborhood was much more ethnically diverse and felt that they had more knowledge of ethnic values than the neighborhood leaders.

Clergy also were more sensitive to, or knowledgeable of, the problems facing the four specific population groups than most of the other interview groups. Although the clergy were familiar with problems, they indicated little knowledge of resources outside the church to address those problems. Most other interview groups, particularly in Milwaukee, believe that the clergy play a very significant helping role, but no other interview group believes that the role of the clergy is as important as the clergy themselves perceive it to be. This difference has led to efforts to provide opportunities for clergy to engage in these potential roles.

Clergy and neighborhood leaders gave similar responses in ranking the neighborhood as a place to live and designating important community issues; natural helpers' and human service workers' responses to the same questions also tended to parallel one another. These two sets of paired groups also identified the same resources as helpful for problems. The similarities in these groups may arise from the similarities of their particular helping roles: Natural helpers and human service professionals primarily care for individuals; the clergy and the neighborhood leaders are mostly men involved in broader community roles.

A critical finding about physicians and pharmacists is that very high percentages of both report that people come to them for help with personal problems and that they refer people to other services. This is consistent with earlier studies of physicians' gatekeeping roles. In Milwaukee in particular, physicians are very clearly the professionals that many other lay and professional helpers rely on for advice. Physicians and pharmacists showed a low level of interest in and knowledge about natural helpers in both cities, perhaps reflecting their lack of integration into the lay helping network, or perhaps indicating reservations about the potential utility of such helpers. One task emerging from the data was the necessity to link primary health care providers (family doctors) and the social and mental health networks.

School personnel seemed to be another unintegrated and isolated helper group. They had the least knowledge about major community issues identified by other helpers and leaders. In Milwaukee, they had the highest "don't know/no response" percentages, and in both cities they cited the smallest number of issues per interviewee. In both cities, they specified primarily issues relevant to the schools, such as integration and busing. In Baltimore, they exhibited the least knowledge of problems of three out of the four population groups. In both cities, they indicated least knowledge about the role of natural helpers in the neighborhoods.

As might be expected, all interview groups tended to define situations according to their own experiences and vantage points, or through their own "colored glasses." For instance, the frequency with which people cited problems was related to the kind of problems they encounter in their roles. Each group consistently cited themselves or resources from their own lay or professional network as "most helpful." School personnel, for instance, cited the school as most helpful for the problems of teens. They reported seeking advice first from other school personnel. Human service agency personnel consistently picked professional agencies as most helpful. Problem recognition and resource definitions are obviously very narrow and circumscribed, an indicator demonstrating lack of linkages among and between helper groups.

POPULATION GROUPS (TEENS, FAMILIES, THE SEPARATED/DIVORCED, AND THE ELDERLY)

Responses to questions about teens were strikingly different from responses about the other population groups. They were also the most diverse. More problems involving teens were cited in both cities that were cited for other population groups. The only real agreement about resources for teens was a conviction that they did not exist. Neighborhood leaders particularly described this lack of resources. Most interviewees, furthermore, saw teens in a rather negative light. They were widely believed to do nothing about their problems and to engage in dysfunctional behavior. This response to problems was rarely cited for the other population groups. Those who did see teens using helping resources reported only a rather scattered usage. Interviewees seemed somewhat mystified by teens. Although they know that teens have a lot of problems and engage in acting-out behavior, they expressed confusion about the best approach to handle these problems, or even whether the appropriate resources exist. Field experience indicates that there are actually few services designed to meet the needs of teens. This is further complicated both by the developmental state of adolescence itself, in which peer group orientations are at their peak, and by the complex legal issues raised in offering services to minors.

The interviewees' perceptions about the problems of families represents a laundry list of the social impingements affecting families across the country. Communication and relationship issues of parent/child/family problems were consistently held primary for each of the interview groups. It is likely that the communication and relationship issue is an outcome of the stress caused by changing family structures and roles.

Whereas interviewees frequently mentioned that people have

financial problems, it was not clear whether they understand the connection between economics, changing family structures, and the resultant family strain. This is borne out in their choice of resources for families. Many interviewees also thought that the Department of Social Services (Public Welfare) was most helpful. Although this resource certainly focuses on the financial component of family problems, it does not really offer a viable solution for anyone except the most desperately poor. Departments of social service rarely have the resources to put into effect the multiple service and multiple network approach needed to address family issues most effectively.

High separation and divorce rates create many one-parent families. Some problems of the separated/divorced are unique to them, but generally their problems parallel those of intact families, only with greater intensity. Both the financial problems and the parent/child/family problems can become severe for the separated/divorced. The most critical findings about this group are that the lay network interviewees showed the highest lack of knowledge in reference to this population group, and that no interview group provided much service to the separated/divorced group. This lack is further accentuated by the fact that this high-risk group exists in both target areas in higher proportions than in the corresponding city and state. Of the two networks, the professional network knew the most about this group, although a large number of professionals did lack knowledge about the problems and resources of the separated/divorced. Professionals possibly know more about the separated/divorced because this group can seek help from professionals with less fear of stigma than from approaching lay helpers, and because social service professionals are one of the only resources for financial difficulties. The gap between the professional and lay network needs to be bridged because the spearated/divorced especially need the support and encouragement of their communities.

Lack of family support seems to be a serious factor affecting problems experienced by the elderly. When the elderly can no longer earn a living and do not have the support of a family, financial problems (including the cost of medical care) and loneliness become more severe. Coping with the mobility and management aspects of health care, and with protection from crime, is difficult without the support of a family or spouse. The elderly often lack family support not only because families live at a distance or children are deceased, but also because families frequently cannot themselves handle the financial burden of the elderly. Neugarten (1974) describes the emergence of a new situation in which increased life expectancies have created families in which couples have dependent children and dependent parents who are expected to live longer than ever. In time past, parents did not live long beyond the time their children began their own families.

The data showed that the lay network interviewees were much more knowledgeable about the elderly than the professional network interviewees. Whereas the separated/divorced seem stigmatized within the lay communities, the problems of the elderly seem to be insufficiently addressed by the professional community. The gap between the lay and professional networks once again needs bridging because families and communities no longer have adequate resources by themselves to care for the elderly. For professional and community helpers to work in tandem to address the needs of the elderly seems a logical conclusion.

GENERAL CONCLUSIONS

Four central themes emerge from the data: community strengths, community needs, community obstacles, and community potentials.

COMMUNITY STRENGTHS

Both the Baltimore and Milwaukee communities have considerable strengths. Community helpers and leaders express generally positive feelings about the neighborhoods they serve. Both communities tend to be stable, having many helpers and leaders who not only live in the neighborhood but who have done so for many years. These positive feelings about the community exist despite the many community issues and problems uncovered in the field survey. The data also show that a strong sense of community pride permeates both communities. Although helpers who do not have positive feelings about their neighborhood would not refuse help to individuals, it is doubtful that they would expend efforts on community activities in behalf of neighborhoods that they regard as unimportant. Lack of pride might indicate that they have little stake in the community. If a community helping network is to be developed, it needs helpers who feel a commitment to the neighborhood. Clearly, this attitudinal prerequisite existed in both target neighborhoods.

There are many lay helpers in both the Baltimore and Milwaukee communities, an important community strength. The data provided conflicting impressions about the significance of the actual helping role of the clergy. Despite this, it was very clear that the clergy, especially the Catholic clergy, possessed major helping potential—especially their availability as helpers. There were a significant number of them and they lived in the community. Their services were convenient, and they had time to get to know community residents and their needs. Clergy also possess special inherent legitimacy as helpers. In the first place, they see helping as a critical part of their overall role; and in the second place, they are regarded highly as helpers by both lay and professional helpers. These positive factors of availability and legitimacy enhanced the potential to expand their helping role. Natural helpers, neighborhood leaders, pharmacists, and physicians were also found to play important helping roles. Lay helpers clearly provide many needed services to community residents. Without the services they provide, professional helping systems would become overloaded, and some community residents would go without any help at all; others would not know where to go or would be afraid to go for help.

A related strength was that, in both communities, residents wanted to take care of their own problems. People felt that community resources could be very important, especially in situations that had not reached serious psychiatric proportions. This was especially clear from the responses to a projective vignette concerning school behavior. Lay interviewees showed a distinct preference for family and other lay resources as appropriate for addressing the problem, suggesting an attitudinal and behavioral predisposition towards preventive activities. Field experience reinforced these data findings. In both communities, numerous individuals and organizations expressed willingness to become involved in community-based efforts.

Lay helpers also seemed quite willing and able to recognize the need for a division of labor. Helpers were clearly able to recognize psychiatric situations when faced with them. In these instances, they felt that mental health professionals were very important. The psychiatric admission rates, family referral rates, and self-referral rates supported this point. There has proven to be a refreshing common sense in the community about high-technology medical intervention; a common sense sometimes wanting among those who write theoretical pieces about neighborhood care to the exclusion of needed specialty care.

Community helpers stated that individuals came to them largely out of trust. It should be pointed out that trust is a critical and necessary factor in the helping process, and thus represents a considerable strength. In psychological terms, help-receiving and help-giving involve relationships. Relationships are in turn based on trust. Trust as a factor was even more important in both of these communities because of the stigma attached to asking for help.

Both communities had strong organizations already at work in the neighborhood. In Milwaukee, they were mostly of a school, ethnic, or fraternal type; in Baltimore, there was more emphasis on neighborhood advocacy organizations. Despite the differences in type, organizations in both areas added to community stability and assisted people in need. Each one was a self-help apparatus or structure already in place. As such, they represented an incipient helping network.

The professional helpers in the community added considerably to community strengths. Professionals also expressed generally positive feelings about the neighborhoods they serve, suggesting that they saw the neighborhoods as positive environments for social interaction and that they were optimistic about them. In common with lay helpers, it is doubtful that professionals who were pessimistic about neighborhood possibilities would be willing to cooperate with community efforts to build integrated helping networks in those communities.

In general, professionals were providing very needed service even though there were gaps in the services that they provided. Preventive services were severely lacking, and certain population groups had either very limited or no services available to them. Yet there was not a total service vacuum. The professional components for a potentially integrated lay/professional helping network already existed for the most part, before our project was initiated. There was also much agreement between lay and professional helpers about which problems existed. The level of agreement was hardly total, and there were differences of opinion about the priority of problems, but lay and professional helpers held many convergent views. This factor suggested the potential for developing partnerships based on shared perceptions.

Professional helpers did seem willing to be involved in the community. They indicated that they belonged to community groups and that community groups used their facilities. This suggested that an incipient relationship already existed among the professionals and the community helpers. The relationships appeared ready for development and direction in the demonstration phases of the project.

One overall strength should also be noted. For almost all problems and for each "at-risk" population group, there seemed to be at least one helping group, lay or professional, that had knowledge about that problem or group and the resources appropriate for the problem or the needs of the group. Development of a coordinated, integrated network system implied that the knowledgeable helping groups could influence and educate the less aware groups. This process would amount to a self-correction mechanism that would limit service gaps and blind spots about "at-risk" groups.

COMMUNITY NEEDS

The data showed that there were also considerable needs in both communities. Changing family structures and financial needs had combined to put stress on both the Baltimore and Milwaukee communities. In terms of family structure, the breakdown of traditional families was the focus of many interrelated problems for all the population groups. In both communities, there were a large number of divorced, widowed, female-headed households with children and aged individuals, all of which are considered to be "at-risk" populations. In addition, males in both communities had needs caused by low-status occupations and difficulties in asking for help. These factors combined to create strong pressures on males in the communities. Many of the above situations stemmed from the changing economic structure in the long run and the current economic situation in the short run. It was not surprising that financial pressures in both communities appeared as a recurring theme, with the Baltimore community under greater stress because of its higher numbers of low-income residents and individuals living in poverty.

The pressures described above created specific "at-risk" groups whose needs tended to go unrecognized. Scrutiny of other population groups and other kinds of data could well reveal additional groups "at-risk," and additional groups lacking services. As indicated in the next section, the needs of many individuals in these communities were ignored because of numerous obstacles involved in the help-seeking and receiving processes.

COMMUNITY OBSTACLES

Within both target neighborhoods, there were many obstacles that prevented individuals from seeking and/or receiving help. Major help-seeking obstacles included: pride or inability to ask for help; not wanting others to know of a problem; and not knowing where to go for help. An interesting finding was that the stigma involved in seeking help was mentioned to a greater degree by professionals than by lay helpers, raising questions about the amount of stigma actually felt by community residents. This is concordant with our earlier studies (Crocetti, Spiro, & Siassi, 1974).

The data revealed fragmentation in helping networks. Fragmentation occurred in two ways. First, the service networks were incomplete; that is, there were some community problems for which there were insufficient services. Second, there were insufficient linkages within the lay and professional helping networks and between the two networks.

The evidence of this fragmentation was apparent in a number of ways. Many helpers and leaders were unaware of the major problems of community residents. While they could identify specific problems if confronted with them, they were unaware of the overall picture. Thus, a helper might know that a particular family was having a specific problem, but that helper would not know whether that same problem affected many other families in the neighborhood. Many lay and professional helpers indicated an even greater lack of awareness of the networks utilized by community residents to meet their needs. Each interview group looked at problems and needs from its own perspective, which tended to be narrowly-based. Lay helpers were more aware of lay networks than professional helpers were, and vice versa. There was reliance by both the lay and professional network interviewees on only a few resources as helpful for addressing community needs. Not only were professionals unaware of the important roles played by lay helpers, but often lay helpers themselves did not fully appreciate the scope, magnitude, and helpfulness of the services they provided.

The fragmentation of the helping networks caused by each of the above dynamics prevented linkages between and among helpers. This lack of linked helping networks was evident both within networks and between networks. Examples of this would include the Catholic priest in a parish who was unaware of the counseling roles of other Catholic clergy in nearby parishes; or the two administrators of mental health clinics in South East Baltimore who had never met each other despite the fact that they served the same neighborhoods; or the natural helper who was unaware of another helper only a few blocks away who was performing a similar role to hers. On an internetwork level, the general lack of awareness by lay and professional helpers of mutual and/or complementary roles prevented any effective linking of services.

Linkages were also prevented by professionals being unaware of community values in regard to helping. Lay helpers frequently defined certain problem situations in the study as nonpsychiatric, and in those situations preferred to make use of community helping resources (i.e., the family, clergy, etc). Professionals, on the other hand, defined the same situation as one in which psychiatric intervention would be warranted and appropriate. However, if professionals would refer residents to other professionals in situations that lay people regarded as nonpsychiatric, and for which they felt professionals are inappropriate, it would not be likely that the residents would follow through and seek professional help. Professionals' expertise had to be translated into meaningful terms for lay helping networks. Professionals are currently very concerned about the negative effects of labeling. Intervention through lay networks has been found to reduce and frequently eliminate the potential for labeling. In relation to school behavior problems, for example, it is not likely that teens and their families will be stigmatized by attending community-sponsored family life education activities at their local schools.

Fragmentation of services is also caused by the lack of sufficient services to meet community needs. Mental health services in the Baltimore community, for example, were primarily crisis-oriented; in contrast, the Milwaukee community had a comprehensive mental health program considered by some to have been one of the best in the nation. Referrals by SCO in Milwaukee had direct access to Medical College of Wisconsin faculty specialists practicing in a modern physical plant. Despite the dual pressures in Baltimore around financial needs and changing family structures, significant preventive mental health services, such as self-help groups, support services for day-care or displaced homemakers, or family communication workshops, were lacking. Milwaukee had some unique prevention services, such as a 0–3-year-old preschool program and a stress reduction team, but ties to the SCO neighborhood were lacking.

COMMUNITY POTENTIALS

It is evident that the lay communities and the professional communities in both target areas had strengths as well as needs and obstacles that prevented needs from being met. It is ironic that these strengths had not been effectively utilized to overcome the obstacles and therefore to improve ability to meet community needs. This is not a situation peculiar to the Baltimore and Milwaukee communities. Lack of coordination and fragmentation of services have been studied at many levels in many communities. One current answer to these issues has been the development of an integrated service delivery network. However, this strategy has been aimed only at integrating the professional services, to the exclusion or denial of lay helpers' services.

Our data revealed a strong potential for the development of an integrated lay and professional service delivery network. The focus on community strengths showed that incipient networks were already in place and that numerous additional network components were available. Positive community feeling and self-help values were expected to help to catalyze this incipient network into a full helping system. Additionally, the stable and nontransitory nature of the community suggested that an established system would not easily collapse. Network-building efforts in such communities tend to be self-reinforcing and self-generating. Good potential existed for linkages to the professional network because lay helpers recognized the importance of professional services, particularly in relation to serious psychiatric difficulties. There was also a strong potential for complementary linkages by the professional network. The professionals' high regard for the neighborhood, their beginning involvement in communities (community organization memberships, etc), their willingness to provide convenient services, and their ability to agree, for the most part, with lay helpers about the definition of problems, all suggested that professionals could develop partnerships with lay helpers. The creation of two fully integrated helping systems, because of the linkages between them, would be fully complementary and highly coordinated.

These first steps provided diagnostic data, which the respective community organizations could process. Shared perceptions of needs and resources were identified so that a process of neighborhood consensus building could begin. Chapters 9 and 10 describe the process of developing demonstration programs in each city based on the initial data findings.

CHAPTER 9

The Model in Action—Baltimore

THE COMMUNITY

South East Baltimore is a community known throughout the city for its ethnic diversity. People of Polish, Czechoslovakian, Russian, German, Greek, and Italian origin are all found here. In 1970, over 99,000 people—comprising 11% of the city's population—lived in South East, most of them in well-kept rowhouses, some of which date back to the late eighteenth century.

The community is bounded to the east by the city line, to the west by Fallsway, to the north by Madison Street, and to the south by Baltimore's important harbor. Most of the South East is residential, although the area adjacent to the harbor is taken up by industry. Three large commercial strips, despite a substantial loss of consumer dollars to suburban shopping areas, have survived. Three large medical facilities serve the area: Baltimore City Hospital in the East Highlandtown neighborhood; the famous Johns Hopkins University Hospital in the Broadway area; and the smaller Church Home Hospital. The decreasing number of physicians in private practice and the scarcity of local pharmacists in the South East have created significant dependence for care by residents on these health institutions. A multitude of small church parishes, which once served small, close-knit ethnic communities, still exist, even though many parishioners have long since moved to the suburbs.

South Easts's population is older and poorer than most communities. Fully 25% of South Easts's residents are over 60, 30% of the residents over age 65 live in poverty, and almost 30% of the children under 19 live in poverty. The area's incomes are lower than national averages: 40% of South East's population earns less than the standard for a low-budget family of four. Once wage earners reach a higher level of income, they tend to move elsewhere.

The first draft of this chapter was written by Joseph Coffey.

Youth under age 19 comprise 33% of South East's population. A high percentage of them live in single-parent families. One-third of South East families are headed by women. The percentage of youth who leave high school before grade completed is higher than the national average, and the average school grade completed is lower. About 7,000 schoolage youth are out of school and unemployed. Juvenile delinquency has been on the increase in recent years.

The percentage of nonwhite population has remained constant at 12% over the past two decades. The negligible change in the area's social composition, despite complete changes in surrounding areas, is a good indication of the stable nature of the South East community. People have not panicked in the face of real estate exploitation, block-busting, or redlining. Integration to a certain degree has not been intolerable. Social stability has contributed to an economic stability. Few people have not sold their homes or moved for fear of a "changing neighborhood"; problems often characteristic of rapidly changing neighborhoods have not been exhibited here. Stability in population composition indicates that social services may be adequately planned and implemented, and assessed without disruption in continuity of services by a changing constituency.

A high percentage of home owners is usually a reliable indicator of neighborhood stability. South East Baltimore has a lower rate of home ownership than the national average, but its rate of over 50% has remained fairly constant since 1950. There seems to be no indication that the rate of home ownership in the area will decrease in the near future. Recent neighborhood revitalization programs may even help to increase the percentage of home owners.

The professional mental health service system serving the South East population principally consists of two state-funded community mental health centers that are based in the two large urban hospitals located on the northern and eastern fringes of the community. These two centers receive most referrals of local residents needing psychiatric assistance. Many of these referrals come through the hospitals' emergency rooms. Residents appeared to connect with a professional service primarily in times of crisis and emergency. The two mental health centers coordinate their services with alcohol, drug, social work, and aftercare divisions within each of the hospitals. In addition, a number of public and private agencies dealing with drugs, alcohol, mental health, day-care, youth, senior citizens, and the poor or near-poor serve the community in piecemeal fashion. Little identifiable community outreach occurred in any of the established services at the beginning of the Neighborhood and Family Services Project, although in the 1960s the Johns Hopkins University Hospital had developed a very active program under the leadership of one of the authors (Herzl Spiro). In the early 1970s, this program had closed down.

THE SPONSORING ORGANIZATION—SOUTH EAST COMMUNITY ORGANIZATION, INC. (SECO)

The South East Community Organization is an umbrella type group of approximately 75 neighborhood improvement associations, block clubs, tenant councils, school PTAs, and churches. SECO officially came into being in April of 1971, when its first Annual Congress was held. It was the culmination of the efforts of several neighborhood groups that had been working together since the late 1960s to prevent a federally funded expressway from running through the South East community.

Most of SECO's record of achievements at the neighborhood level has actually been the work of its constituent member groups. Its function has been to support neighborhood leaders and encourage their efforts to provide community organization assistance, and in some instances to secure funds that have made projects and programs possible.

SECO is governed by a Senate. Each member group sends one representative (Senator) to the monthly Senate meetings that determine SECO policy. The Annual Meeting, or Congress, elects community officers to SECO and selects issues the organization will address in the next year. SECO's Executive Committee consists of its officers, Senators-at-large, and representatives of its various committees and task forces. The Executive Committee plans the agenda for Senate meetings and manages organizational business between monthly Senate meetings. In the summer of 1973, SECO began its first social service program, the Youth Diversion Project, in which local young people in legal difficulties were referred to SECO for counselling and community support services. This component of SECO has expanded to include a program to develop services for teenage soft-drug abusers, a tutoring service, development of recreational facilities, and a program to secure jobs for youth.

In the autumn of 1974, the SECO Senate voted to form South East Development, Inc., a subsidiary corporation, to plan, finance, and manage economic and physical development projects. Its activities have included programs to increase home ownership and to encourage commercial revitalization and industrial development.

In 1975, a SECO Planning Component was formed to assist SECO to give direction to South East Development. The Planning Component has since expanded to explore funding resources, to develop mental health services, to provide services to the aged, and to do long-term planning for SECO.

Recently, the SECO Senate has organized a Human Services Component to develop a broad-based community constituency for human service issues and to give community direction to human service programs. Our project in SECO was part of the Human Services Component. The project was responsible to the SECO Human Services Board, which consisted of community representatives from each of the human service programs.

In Spring of 1976, SECO signed a contractual agreement with National Center for Urban Ethnic Affairs to carry out the Neighborhood and Family Services Project. For the first two years, $19,000 per year was provided for employment of a project coordinator; in the second two years, $25,000 per year was allotted and an additional staff person was employed. In view of the very large sums of money expended on putative "community" mental health programs, these relatively low costs may be of interest to planning bodies. The project coordinator hired by SECO was a social worker who had worked for SECO for two years in various organizing capacities. He had an Italian background and he understood ethnic communities and neighborhood life. He was well liked, respected, and trusted by neighborhood residents. SECO set up a community board (later called the Neighborhood and Family Services Task Force) to represent the community, to oversee the project, and to give direction to staff. The grant shifted to the University of Southern California in 1977 when the senior author became Director of its Public Affairs Center in Washington, D.C.

A unique partnership arrangement was developed between SECO and the University of Southern California (USC) in the conduct of the project. SECO's previous experience with research and demonstration projects had been with the National Center for Urban Ethnic Affairs (NCUEA), under whose auspices SECO received a number of subcontracts. While each of these subcontracts was monitored by NCUEA, SECO conducted each project independently with only limited assistance and direction from NCUEA. USC staff felt that the nature of the mental health project, with its far-reaching and complicated objectives, required a closer working partnership. Through this partnership effort, very close and productive working relationships were developed between the SECO and USC project staff.

DEVELOPMENT OF THE COMMUNITY TASK FORCE

Before the Community Task Force was formed in Spring 1976, SECO selected four community leaders to oversee SECO staff efforts in the organization of a representative Task Force. The organizer began recruitment by talking individually and informally to as many residents as possible. As the philosophy of the project was explained, mental health was discussed within the context of "problems in living." The organizer emphasized the importance of community residents defining their own needs and giving shape and direction to the project. Residents were told that they would decide which demonstration projects to implement; that mental health and human service professionals would be recruited to assist the residents in their work; and that staff would provide support, organizational assistance, and technical know-how to the Task Force members.

A dialogue was encouraged among the entire Task Force as new members joined during the 3-month organizing period. A feeling of a "family" soon developed. Since it was felt that life experiences and knowledge of the community by community residents had qualified them to select neighborhood projects, it followed logically that anything anyone said at a meeting ought to be considered worthwhile and carefully considered. This feeling enhanced the cohesiveness of the Task Force during the project. Most members participated throughout the entire course of the Task Force's 3½-year existence. Although the project officially terminated on February 28, 1980, the Task Force continues today and is flourishing.

Too often in classical community organizing strategies, the needs of individuals for support, recognition, and acceptance are unconsciously overlooked in the emphasis on issues, whether it is over a vacant house, street crime, or another matter. The goal of empowering community residents required the development of a "process" for strengthening helping networks in the neighborhood and linking those networks with professional services. This process of network building, by definition, focused on the development of individuals and paid significant attention to individual needs.

Prior to the existence of this Task Force, SECO had been unsuccessful in maintaining task forces for human services longer than a few months. The organization of human service task forces requires much planning, as opposed to action. In organizations like SECO, which are focused on community action to address identified needs, it becomes increasingly difficult to keep residents involved in planning over a long period of time.

We were able to keep the Task Force going through long phases of needs assessment, problem identification, and program development because of emphasis on process issues and group maintenance, as well as task needs. A strong, healthy group process evolved within the Task Force, which fostered active participation by all group members. This kind of a process within a human service group is essential, not only for long-term cohesion of a group, but also to enable the development of more effective human service programs. A task force such as the Neighborhood and Family Services Task Force is qualified to do more than review research results. Task Force members can provide significant input into the implications of the research results. If the research, for example, says that elderly people are lonely and shut-in, then what are the particulars that make this true in South East Baltimore? Answers can best be articulated by involved, motivated residents who know the area and the people and feel confident about expressing their views. Their analysis is as important a part of the research as data gathering.

Task Force members did not want to become identified, or perhaps stigmatized, as a mental health/illness group; they preferred not to limit themselves to the development of traditional mental health services alone. One Task Force member, an experienced and knowledgeable natural helper in the community, suggested that the group call themselves the Neighborhood and Family Services Task Force to project this image of their function. Other Task Force members agreed; the name was soon adopted for the entire two-city project.

MEMBERSHIP

After several months, the SECO Task Force grew to 20 members. Members were all residents of the area. They were a blend of community leaders, natural helpers, former patients, and ordinary citizens concerned with mental health and family issues. Since the sponsorship of SECO, which represented the leadership of the community, already had conferred legitimacy in recruiting Task Force members, the next aim was to involve grassroots residents, as opposed to established, well-known community leaders. The Task Force ultimately became a combination of established leaders and other individuals who were not otherwise involved actively in community-wide activities. Many Task Force members had limited formal education.

A brief description of a few Task Force members will help give a "flavor" to the group.

Mrs. M. is in her 60s and lives with her divorced daughter and two grandchildren. She has lived in South East Baltimore for over 30 years and has been active in community work in her neighborhood for the past 10 years. She is a very active natural helper, well known and regarded by people on her block and in her neighborhood. She likes to get involved with people and lend her support and help. She gets satisfaction showing other residents how to be effective and to get things done. Mrs. M. enjoys opening her home to people, making a dinner for someone she works with or just someone who needs a meal. Her kitchen is sometimes busier than an agency waiting room. She would say she is just a "friend."

When politicians, agency professionals, clergy, or others want an insight into her neighborhood, they contact Mrs. M. She is very proud of the network she has developed. Her network is her power and she uses it very effectively. She has been a very active member of the Task Force, involved in virtually all Task Force activities, especially bringing new residents into projects. She is the "mother" of the SECO Hotline, an information, referral, and counseling service established by the Task Force.

Sr. S. is in her 40s and belongs to an order of nuns, the Sisters of Notre Dame De Namur. She is a former French teacher and principal of a parochial high school. Several months before our project began, she founded and organized, together with another nun, the Julie Community Center in South East Baltimore. Her work is dedicated to empowering neighborhood residents, especially in the health field. She has organized and conducted several health education programs that affirm the power individuals have in taking responsibility for their own health. She works well with both community residents and professionals. Professionals are involved in Julie Community Center as resource specialists.

Similarities in philosophy between the Task Force and Julie Community Center enabled the two to cosponsor several programs. Consequently, community networks were strengthened without the Task Force going into competition with an existing group. Sr. S., a particularly effective member of the Task Force, became a group facilitator working conscientiously and skillfully to enhance participation by all Task Force members.

Mrs. L. is in her 60s and is a widow who currently lives alone in the same South East Baltimore neighborhood where she has lived since childhood. She has raised a large family, but all of her children have moved to the suburbs. Despite their invitations to live with them, she refuses to leave the neighborhood she loves. Her husband died 10 years ago after a long illness that had left him bedridden. Caring for him during his illness, she became self-sufficient. A gregarious, outgoing woman, she loves people. Before her husband's illness, she would sell "snowballs" (flavored ice) and then sandwiches from her livingroom window in Fells Point. Kids gathered there from all over the neighborhood, and her house soon became known as "Lil's Sub Shop."

Mrs. L. adapted her life experiences very usefully to the Task Force. Her love of cooking stimulated her to plan and organize several very successful fund-raising dinners. As treasurer, she organized various ongoing fund-raising activities. She helped to establish such Task Force projects as "Peace at Sundown" (visiting relatives of deceased hospital patients) and "CHEN" (a mental health education network). Although she and Mrs. M. were good friends, they often got into friendly disputes. Mrs. L. felt Task Force activities ought to raise money, but Mrs. M. didn't want the cost to discourage people from attending programs.

Mrs. D. is in her 60s and is a former psychiatric patient whose husband also had been in treatment. When the project began, the Baltimore Mental Health Association provided the names of several of its members who lived in South East Baltimore. Mrs. D. was approached by staff and agreed to join the Task Force. She firmly believes in speaking out about mental health problems to reduce the stigma associated with seeking and receiving help. She often cited her own life experiences and strongly advocated improvements in mental health programs and the expansion of mental health education efforts. Her ideas and recommendations carried considerable weight in the Task Force because of her personal experiences. Her work experience at the Johns Hopkins University Hospital Resource Development Office was of invaluable assistance to the staff in preparing funding proposals.

Mrs. T. is a 30-year neighborhood resident in her mid-60s who has a mentally retarded teenage son. Her husband is physically disabled. Active in support of the center for the retarded, which her son attends, she contributed substantial knowledge and insight about services for the mentally impaired and the elderly to the Task Force proceedings.

Miss H. one of the youngest Task Force members, is a woman in her mid-20s who is a professional counselor for disturbed teens. She was born and raised in South East Baltimore and gets on well with older people. She has been both a facilitator for the group and, on occasion, a resource person. She designed a solid training program for volunteers participating in a crisis hotline.

Mr. O. a 34-year-old accountant, was the Task Force joker. His sharp, but never unkind, wit added fun, energy, and enthusiasm to Task Force sessions. Mr. O. grew up in South East and had a reputation for extending himself to aid the elderly and youth.

STRUCTURE

After almost a year of operation, the Task Force began to discuss the need for a more permanent structure, that is, officers. The impetus for this discussion came from the staff, who were used to working through established community leadership. Such a pattern, as the staff came to realize, was neither appropriate nor desirable for the Task Force. At a meeting in February, 1978, Sr. S. remarked that "in many groups the control is in the hands of a few people. Our group has worked just the opposite. We've all had an equal say and we've operated under the assumption that what everyone says is important. We all have the same goal and we all have a great deal of mutual respect for each other." Everyone agreed that to set up a hierarchial structure with officers meant destroying the group's cohesiveness and special rapport. The group settled instead on this structure: (1) an agenda planning committee; (2) a rotating chairperson; (3) two financial coordinators; (4) two communications coordinators (one for communications within the group, one to represent the group to the outside community); (5) a recorder (secretary); and (6) a historian ("to keep us honest to our roots and philosophy"). The historian would function as a "superego" for the group.

At each monthly Task Force meeting, volunteers would be asked to serve as chairperson and to meet in advance to formulate an agenda for the next regular session. Although this form of rotating chair and planning committee has not worked for other SECO groups, it succeeded with the cohesive Task Force and, in fact, increased commitment. Less educated members of the group, supported by others with greater organizational experience, were able to serve as effective planners and chairmen, a source of special satisfaction to all concerned.

After the Task Force had functioned for three years, it began to prepare for the ending of federal funding and the subsequent reduction in staff support for the Task Force. At a Task Force meeting in April, 1979, it becme clear that while group members understood that the staff did a lot for them, they overlooked the most important staff contributions, responsibilities they might have to assume themselves when their funding ended.

In a process as educational to staff as to Task Force members, staff members presented to the group a list of their "task" and "maintenance" functions. Task functions included: making announcements at meetings; coordinating work with the rest of SECO; researching funding sources and writing grant proposals; writing budget reports; helping to plan agendas; and coordinating commitee work. Group maintenance

functions performed by staff included: encouraging people to be supportive of one another; listening well at meetings to what people were
saying; trying to learn as much as possible from people you were working with; developing flexibility in planning; and helping people to
accomplish their goals by providing technical assistance and personal
support. After considerable discussion of these functions, ways in
which group members could gradually take over certain staff functions
were planned. No major decisions were reached at the initial meeting,
but it paved the way for subsequent discussions and decision making.
Because the matter was broached fully a year before funding ended,
groundwork was laid for institutionalization of the Task Force and its
programs.

FORMATION OF THE PROFESSIONAL ADVISORY COMMITTEE

If the project was to succeed, professional input was needed from
the human service agencies in each target community. Thus the Baltimore Professional Advisory Committee came into being in November,
1976. Its purposes: to keep human service agencies informed about
project status and activities; to secure assistance from agencies in data
gathering; to help develop relationships with agencies that might sponsor demonstration services; to provide professional assistance and ideas
to the Neighborhood Task Force in developing demonstration programs; and to develop and strengthen cohesiveness within the professional helping network.

The Committee began with approximately 15 members, consisting
generally of professional persons, mostly from middle management and
supervisory staff. It has met quarterly since then. Like the Neighborhood Task Force, the Professional Advisory Committee (PAC) significantly expanded its membership during the first project year. Initially,
agency professionals who participated in the project committed themselves only to attend quarterly meetings of the PAC. After the first year,
though, many PAC members were also participating on Task Force
Committees to help plan demonstration projects.

During the first project year, the Task Force and Professional Advisory Committee were kept separate from each other. The initial decision to keep the Task Force and Professional Advisory Committee separate at first was made by project staff. When the project began, we had
hypotheses and assumptions, but neither a fully developed intervention
model nor a set of strategies. We were "winging it," developing our

plans and strategies as we went along. Therefore, we wanted to keep things as simple and uncomplicated as possible in the first year of the project. Keeping the two groups apart was consonant with this plan. We were also afraid that the professionals would "run over" the community residents. We wanted sufficient time for building the capacity of residents to grapple with mental health issues and interact with professionals.

Membership

The PAC members were a varied, interesting group, as can be seen by three brief descriptions below. They enjoyed meeting one another—many for the first time.

Jane S. emerged as one of the PAC leaders. She was deputy director of the Visiting Nurses Association. Jane worked her way up the professional scale, first as a visiting nurse in South East, then as an administrator in VNA. Her approach combined sensitivity to the needs of area residents with eagerness and skill as a "doer" and coordinator. She was good at recognizing potential to coordinate services as well as to initiate new projects. Her vision of the future often guided PAC planning.

Louis M., director of a residential alcoholism treatment center, sees himself as a maverick, pushing for bold innovative programming. He is action-oriented, always urging other PAC members to move more quickly on tasks. His dedication to raising public consciousness about alcoholism is "up front" and clear. He promoted the PAC and its coordinating efforts enthusiastically.

Wanda K., in her 20s, serious-minded, and popular with area residents, was representative to the PAC of the South East Mayor's Station. In her task of responding to residents' special problems, she had invaluable know-how about the inside workings of the professional helping system and its impact on residents. She was responsive to the concept of coordinating services.

Professional and Community Roles

Before PAC members joined the Task Force committees, Task Force members spent considerable time at one of their regular meetings in August, 1977, discussing their relationship with professionals. Sr. S. remarked to group members that,

> In the beginning our group decided we would do as much as possible by ourselves without asking professionals to help. We did this because we didn't want professionals telling us what to do. Now that we have gained

> strength as a group, and have accomplished a great deal, we are in a position
> to tell the agencies how we would like them to help us with out projects.

Task Force members agreed that their group had accomplished a
lot and had worked well together. Comments included "We've done a
lot with very little, just by ourselves," and "It's good we're able to work
together as one big family; we get more done." The consensus of the
discussion that followed was that Task Force members could identify
needs in the community without the help of professionals; but when it
came to providing service to take care of those needs, it was both necessary and helpful to work with professionals. There was concern
expressed, however, that the Task Force should not be "railroaded" by
professionals who are pressed to meet deadlines and agency goals that
may not always be in the community's best interest.

Aware of these concerns, the project staff set up a process in which
the professionals did not dominate the process of planning the demonstration programs through the joint working committees.

This effort has been successful. Professionals involved with the
project have been, for the most part, very conscious about letting the
community articulate its own needs and desires. To reduce any intim-
idation by professionals that the residents might feel, and to prevent
residents from deferring unnecessarily to professional expertise, Task
Force committees were initially organized with only residents as members. Only after the committees had completed a significant amount of
brainstorming and planning were professionals invited to join the committees. This ensured the desired community-directed, agency-sup-
ported process. In addition, staff worked individually with identified
professionals who were likely to be unaware or insensitive to these special goals and needs. This process offered an advantage to professionals
whose schedules were often busy—they had fewer meetings to attend
and they were usually asked for specific input on programs. Mutual
respect, and often friendship, developed over time between agency
professionals and Task Force members. Certainly these relationships
enhanced the planning and implementation of demonstration programs. Agency professionals and community residents developed a better understanding of each other's skills and resources, and in the process, many stereotypes held by each group were dissolved.

ACTION RESEARCH

Both the Task Force and Professional Advisory Committee provided significant input into the development and implementation of the

research design and in the analysis of the research data. The Task Force gave project staff suggestions on questions to include in the community interviews, as well as assistance in the development of lists of people to interview. They advised interviewers on the best ways to approach individuals. They also employed their personal contacts to encourage people to be receptive to the interviewers. Refusal rates for the interviews were significantly below the national average, thanks to these efforts. Members of the PAC were also extremely helpful in suggesting names of persons to be interviewed, securing necessary clearances for interviews in their agencies, and providing social indicator and agency ethnicity data for us.

The Task Force was deeply involved in the analysis of the data findings. The first data available to the Task Force were preliminary analyses of approximately 20 variables from 130 interviews of clergy, neighborhood leaders, and human service agency staff. This material was discussed at several Task Force meetings. Prior to looking at any data, Task Force members would hold a brainstorming session, which would focus on their own views of needs in the community and on possible programs to address those needs. After reviewing the data, a similar exercise was repeated and comparisons were made.

The Task Force members enjoyed this process, but felt that they needed more time than part of their regular meeting agenda to review data. A half-day workshop was arranged to examine the data in detail in the context of three basic questions: What are the problems? Where do people go for help? and, What are the obstacles to seeking and receiving help?

In preparing for the workshop, staff spent several days reviewing the voluminous data collected. The community leader and helper survey alone contained over 300 variables. This process was at first overwhelming. There was a serious problem of data "overload." How were we ever going to understand and work with so much information? We made a conscious decision to separate our analysis into research and program development functions. For program development, we would do a nonstatistical examination of information that would assist us in developing intervention programs. At a later point (which turned out to be 12 months later), we planned to examine the data statistically and in much greater depth for research purposes (our subsequent statistical analysis led to the publication of a 300-page data report of the community helper and leader survey). Decisions about variables to present at the workshop were made by staff. Once particular variables were selected, raw data in tabular form with numbers and percentages were put on huge sheets of newsprint covering the entire walls of the work-

shop room for participants to review. Staff made no summary statements or interpretations of findings.

The workshop was facilitated by a Task Force member, Sr. S., who
was a skilled group leader, well-liked and respected by Task Force
members. The examination of the data at the workshop generated a tremendous amount of energy from Task Force members. They looked at
the results and, in a dialogue with each other and with staff, began to
seek explanations behind the findings (e.g., why did people say that
teenagers had nothing to do? Why was alcoholism a problem?). At the
end of the day, Sr. S. helped group members evaluate the information
they had reviewed. They were asked what surprised them most about
the findings, what was most interesting, and what seemed most important. These questions helped the group to develop some overall statements about the data.

Some of.these statements were: (1) that families and their breakdown was the principal locus of interrelated problems for all population groups in the South East Baltimore community; (2) that a network
of helping systems was needed to provide supports to the family,
whether that family was single, two-parent, or elderly; (3) that the present helping system was fragmented and therefore often unsuccessful
and not useful; (4) that fragmentation among community helpers, as
well as between professional and community helpers, was a major
obstacle to people seeking help, and that this condition made "pride"
and "privacy" take precedence over help-seeking; (5) that people were
not making use of the many strengths that did exist within their community; and (6) that support-system building needed to begin on a
neighborhood level within the community itself.

Shortly after the Task Force workshop, members of the Professional Advisory Committee examined the same data findings in the
context of the same three basic questions, focusing on problems,
resources, and networks. The professionals reacted to the data similarly
to the community residents. Ensuing discussion focused on how, in light
of the research findings, professional agencies could improve their
delivery of services. There was considerable interest expressed at this
point by the professionals who wanted to become involved in the planning of intervention programs. The examination of the data assisted the
process of building a sense of community and identity among the
human service agencies serving South East Baltimore. Agency professionals began to see, many for the first time, the *total* needs of the community, instead of merely focusing on the needs of the "problem" or
specialized population groups they served.

Several issues pertaining to the action research process need to be addressed here. First, the data were examined for program planning and development purposes, not principally for the purposes of research. The findings were used to stimulate group reaction and brainstorming sessions. More data were collected and analyzed in this process than are available to most agencies when they develop new programs. One purpose in interviewing so many community leaders and helpers was that we wanted to be able to go back to them to share what we had learned through their comments, and then try to involve them in the demonstration program planning. Thus, the rationale for the number of interviewees was a programmatic, and not primarily a research, decision.

Second, while the data analysis efforts by the Task Force helped develop their expertise and confidence and showed them how much they really knew about the community, the staff learned even more. Despite the staff's implicit acceptance of the notion of community empowerment, there remained some skepticism about the ability of community residents, many of whom had no more than an eighth grade education, to be able to examine and understand data complex enough to frighten many professionals. After the data review at the Task Force meetings, and subsequently at the Task Force workshop, such staff skepticism vanished. In fact, at a subsequent Task Force meeting attended by several members of the Professional Advisory Committee, one Task Force member busily paged through her data book to find evidence supporting a particular viewpoint raised by one of the agency professionals. If all professionals were so comfortable with research data, the delivery of human services might conceivably proceed more scientifically.

DEVELOPMENT OF DEMONSTRATION PROGRAMS

The process of reflection and dialogue experienced by Task Force members in looking at the research findings became an important and pervading dynamic throughout the life of this group. As we have seen, the Task Force felt that the family should be the focus for intervention. But how should the intervention work? The grant gave the group tremendous flexibility in deciding how to act; there were no rigid guidelines from the funding source. This freedom made it somewhat difficult for the group to settle in its approach at first, but in the long run it led to greater community ownership and commitment to the project.

The Task Force decided next to draw up guidelines to assist them in formulating demonstration programs. Those precepts were (in their own words):

- Community support of all programs.
- Community control of all programs.
- Community definition of problems that the programs will deal with.
- All programs to deal with problems related to mental health.
- Program to use community helping networks.
- The program to bring about more communication among community helpers and between community helpers and professional agencies.
- The program will make a service easier to get or easier to ask for.

In articulating a firm set of criteria for program development, residents had been able to verbalize their own philosophy for working within their community. This philosophy, and the subsequent mode of operation, differentiated the Task Force from all other groups under SECO's umbrella, and, in fact, all other groups in the community at large.

As a next step, the Task Force spent an entire meeting expressing their individual "dreams for families in the community." Each member was asked to state his/her dream, and each was written on newsprint and posted on the wall. The following dreams, which were accepted by a consensus of the group as representative of the thinking of the entire group, included (in the words of the Task Force):

- Neighborhoods could become like extended families.
- Children need spiritual guidance.
- Need for activities that families, parents, and children could do together; for example, recreation.
- Families need to try and understand one another; there must be communication between families.
- Helpers should know of other helpers who help people so they can work together.
- Families have resources for helping people or know where they can get help.
- Need to accept all different kinds of families, young, old, one-parent, or two-parent families.
- Families need to set their own goals for themselves and not follow goals of others.

- Families need to have trust within their families and with other families.
- People need to accept that it's okay to have problems and need help.

The beauty of this dreaming was that it put the formal program-planning process into a context and vocabulary that all Task Force members could understand. The group completed the final step in the initial planning process by developing concrete program ideas that would: achieve the dreams articulated in earlier meetings; meet the needs identified in the research; and be within their own guidelines for creating demonstration programs. Some of the residents' program ideas included (again, in their own words):

- A series of talks on families to groups throughout SECO.
- Neighborhood associations should get involved with family problems.
- Hotline.
- Need to form a "Friends of Families" organization.
- Have "Problems Workshop" to talk about problems.
- Have a "Neighborhood and Family Day," possibly in Patterson Park, but must be careful not to exclude poor. (This can broaden our base in a nonthreatening way. The neighborhood can be seen as a family. We can talk about our ideas and also have speakers. Members of our group can mingle with others, meet people, and let them know they can get help if they have problems. There can also be literature available on the Task Force and on professional agencies in the community.)
- A program to bring neighborhood leaders together and train neighborhood advocates.

The idea for a "Neighborhood and Family Day Picnic" was the most popular, and Task Force members decided to develop this immediately. This first project led to many others over the next three years, including: Hotline, Referral Directory, Clergy–Agency–Community Seminars, Case Study/Brown Bag Luncheons, Council of Human Service Providers, Peace at Sundown Program, and CHEN. CHEN's activities have included: a babysitting cooperative for young mothers; bus trips for the elderly and shut-ins; and a series of workshops on stress.

Federal funding to SECO for the maintenance of Task Force activities and programs ended in February, 1980, after four years of support, but it appears clear that the project in Baltimore is still thriving. Meetings of the Task Force and its committees are continuing, as are activities such as the Hotline, Case Study/Brown Bag Luncheons, and Clergy–Agency Seminars. The Task Force, however, has left SECO because it felt its work was no longer receiving sufficient support from the umbrella group. It is now meeting actively with the Council of South East Human Service Programs, and the prognosis for its continuance is good.

CHAPTER 10

The Model in Action—Providence and Milwaukee

THE PROVIDENCE PROLOGUE—WHAT WENT WRONG

The two original target cities in our project were Baltimore, Maryland, and Providence, Rhode Island, where we expected to work through existing community organizations. Planning commenced several years before the formal submission of a grant application to NIMH in 1974. In 1972 and 1973, community groups had been contacted to assess potential interest.

Federal Hill in Providence, an almost exclusively Italian working-class neighborhood with 12,000 residents, was a first choice with Neighborhood Organization of Italian-Americans (NOI) as host. By the time grant funding was arranged three years after our initial contact with NOI, the organization had folded. We needed a new host organization.

Staff based in Washington, D.C., traveled to Providence to lay the groundwork. In a single month, three separate two-day trips were made and some 30 meetings were held with representatives of Federal Hill neighborhood groups and with professional agencies there. The mayor of Providence had shown a strong interest in community-based services. Arthur Naparstek (the principal investigator of this funded program) and the mayor had established a good working relationship on a number of other neighborhood related programs. Naparstek served as the project director for a program which was aimed at assisting municipal officials serve moderate and low income communities more effectively. His credibility with the mayor was high. The mayor agreed to appoint a Federal Hill Mental Health Advisory Committee, which would be composed of neighborhood and agency representatives. A local host organization was to receive funds to staff this Advisory Com-

The first draft of the Milwaukee section of this chapter was written by John Andreozzi.

135

mittee, to conduct the research, and to develop the action demonstration programs.

The host organization needed to be located in Federal Hill, and it needed community-wide support. A dual approach was developed, first, to find nominees for the Mental Health Advisory Committee, and second, to secure a host organization to sponsor the project in Federal Hill. Opinions of many persons needed consideration before a host organization could be selected. Eventually 28 persons expressed interest in participating on the Advisory Committee with nine agency representatives, including: Commissioner, Rhode Island Department of Mental Health, Retardation and Hospitals; Planner, Providence Mental Health Center; Epidemiological and Mental Health Consultant, Department of Psychiatry, Brown University; Director, Pupil Personnel Services, Providence Public Schools; representatives of five private social service agencies; two Federal Hill business representatives; and 16 community residents. Agencies seemed so interested in the project that we stopped initiating contact for fear that we would have too many to accommodate on the Advisory Committee.

The community residents we contacted expressed interest but also caution. Many people became uneasy at the mention of "mental health." Staff were asked to change the name of the project to something other than "mental health." In talking with community residents, the name of one neighborhood agency, The Federal Hill House, was often mentioned, always positively. It is a settlement house that has been serving the Italian residents of the area for more than 100 years. Its executive director, a young Italian-American, was initially hesitant about our project; after a number of meetings and the development of a positive relationship with project staff, however, he seemed to want Federal Hill House to serve as sponsor. He felt that many Federal Hill residents refused to go to mental health centers for counseling, and that the agencies in the community did not understand ethnic values and traditions.

Project staff requested that the board of directors of Federal Hill House serve as sponsor for the project. The executive director assured project staff that the meeting of the board to approve such sponsorship would be a mere formality. After all, the Federal Hill House would be receiving money to help improve service delivery to Federal Hill residents, an inherent part of their basic mission. The project director traveled to Providence for the meeting of the board. He arrived in Federal Hill just a few minutes before the meeting for what would be his first contact with board members. The meeting did not go as planned.

The board consisted of approximately 15 middle- and upper-class

Italian males—businessmen, doctors, lawyers, and other professionals. The project director was asked to make a brief presentation about the proposal. As he started to describe its purpose and stated that it would help address mental health problems in Federal Hill, he was interrupted and verbally attacked by a number of Board members. Why was he picking on Federal Hill? What evidence did he have to show that there were mental health problems here? Why was an Italian area chosen? Who invited the project into Federal Hill? The board chairman summed up the feelings of the group when he remarked that the Federal Hill House had been in existence for over 100 years, providing excellent services to the community, and that, "We are afraid that the stigma of mental illness might rub off on our organization." With that, the board refused to act as a local sponsor for the project.

A number of organizational mistakes were made by project staff in Providence. Generalizing from this experience, we learned some valuable lessons that have since been applied to Baltimore and Milwaukee. We learned first of all that the matter of legitimacy is very important in ethnic communities. If one is not invited into a community by community leadership, then legitimacy must be established before any program contracting can be done with other organizations. We should not have attempted to contract with the Federal Hill House until we were sure that board members felt that we had a legitimate reason to be in the community and an appropriate role to play. Second, we learned that a project such as this cannot be organized from Washington on a consultative basis. If project staff had been on-site in Providence, they would not have gone "blind" into the board meeting. Any good organizer, administrator, or political leader knows never to ask an organization to vote on anything until there is some assurance in advance about how the vote will go. With staff commuting from Washington, time was insufficient to develop the necessary "process." Too much attention was focused instead on "product" (in this case, a formal agreement with the Federal Hill House). The development of a process can be slow and requires painstaking attention. Mutual trust must develop, and this in turn requires day-to-day contact by staff who become identified with the neighborhood and are not viewed as outsiders or highly paid Washington consultants. We learned finally that the stigma of mental illness and the fear of labeling remains strong in ethnic communities. An outsider who comes in and talks about mental health problems is suspect. A better strategy would have been to discuss the strengths in ethnic communities, and how these strengths might be utilized to meet identified needs of residents.

With our well-learned lesson behind us, we humbly packed our bags and headed West to Milwaukee where our colleague, Dr. Spiro, who had helped design the original project, had settled. His role as Medical College Chairman of Psychiatry and Director of Psychiatry for Milwaukee County promised to facilitate linkage building. His experience as a social psychologist in community organization and early work in East Baltimore with SECO promised to be useful in developing a new organization. Perhaps what was even more important was his understanding of the need for psychiatrists to remain disengaged and leave room for the community organization specialist to work with the neighborhood process *before* linkages could be formed.

THE MODEL IN ACTION—MILWAUKEE

THE COMMUNITY

The area selected on Milwaukee's Southside is composed of some 22 census tracts. This area in 1975 had a population of 66,074, down some 10% from the 1970 figure of 73,351. Over 99% of the population is white, and 16% of this total is first- or second-generation Polish-American, while 8% is German. Over 32% of the area's population is of foreign stock (i.e., foreign-born, or at least one foreign-born parent).

The median income for families and individuals in the SCO area is higher than that for both the city of Milwaukee and the United States. Only 7% of SCO residents are in poverty; this is one-half of the national rate. The median school years completed are 10.6, fewer than in the city of Milwaukee or in the nation. Population in the SCO area tends to be older than for that of Milwaukee or the nation. It is a stable population with less than one-fifth defined as recently moved (in the previous 5 years).

There are 18 Catholic and two Eastern Orthodox churches in the area. The 19 Protestant churches in the area are mostly smaller in size than the Catholic parishes, and often the former draw parishioners from outside of the area. The population is heavily Catholic, Polish, and working class. Census data indicate that the northern section of the target area is less prosperous and more transitional. Latinos from the near Southside and rural whites are slowly moving there. This target area is probably one of the most, if not the most, visible ethnic communities in the city; that is, not only are there many ethnics in the area, but their institutions and customs are very visible.

The SCO area is characterized by a large number of parks and detached two-and-a-half story houses called "Polish flats." Many of these houses were originally one-story homes and were expanded to provide enough room for two generations to live in the same house.

In or adjacent to the target area are 23 public schools—17 elementary, 3 junior high, and 3 high schools. There are 6 Lutheran elementary schools in the area and 21 Catholic schools, one of the latter a high school. The churches are probably the most important institutions in the area.

There is a Community Mental Health Center serving the Southside, one of seven in Milwaukee County. The CMHC has outreach centers, which serve the target area. A private agency, Catholic Social Services (CSS), until recently operated a "pilot project" in one of the area parishes, offering a range of counseling and advocacy services geared to the Polish community. The existence of the CSS program at the start of our efforts was very helpful because it provided a limited "model" for what we were trying to accomplish. The CSS project ended because of lack of clients; this resulted chiefly because the program failed to engage in outreach activities with neighborhood helpers and leaders. There are many other counseling services in the area, but they are located in or adjacent to the heavily Latino community, and are thus less accessible or attractive to the South Community Organization area. There are also private hospitals near the community that have psychiatric units and services.

ORGANIZATION AND DEVELOPMENT OF THE SPONSORING ORGANIZATION

In Milwaukee, no community organization existed that represented the entire Southside. The first step, here, was to hire a community organizer to form a community organization that could act as a local sponsor for the project. This was a slow and time-consuming process, but absolutely essential to the success of the project.

To achieve community legitimacy it was necessary to locate key community and institutional leadership and solicit their support and endorsement of the project. The Providence experience behind us, we proceeded carefully and cautiously. Since we had not been invited into the community and we didn't have even a single community contact, the issue of community legitimacy was critical. In Baltimore, we could subcontract with an existing neighborhood-based organization that already had community legitimacy; in Milwaukee, we started from scratch. The Milwaukee experience may be more comparable to other parts of the country.

The organizer hired for the project was a sociologist with previous community organizing experience on the East Side of Milwaukee. He was Italian, with pride in his working-class background. The combination of his professional background, community organizing experience, and ethnic identification made him an ideal candidate for the difficult task of gaining entry and developing an organization in Milwaukee's Southside.

The initial strategy in Milwaukee was to learn slowly about the Southside, with special emphasis on discovering the crucial leaders and the key institutions in the community. The organizer, who was unfamiliar with the Southside community, met with people he knew who were from the area and who provided him with names of several key leaders in the Polish community. Interviewing each of these people, he asked them to provide names of other Southsiders who were knowledgeable about their community and who might be interested in the project. Through this "chain" contact technique, the worker spoke with some 70 persons. He gave a general description of the project to each and explained how it would incorporate and build upon the cohesion and strengths of the community. From each interview, he learned more about the leaders, the key institutions, and social networks in the area.

During this initial organizing process, a number of strategies were followed: First, learning from the Providence experience, the organizer stressed that the project would build on the *strengths* in the community; talk of "problems" was minimized. There were indeed valuable, considerable strengths in the community; we were not merely telling people what we thought they wanted to hear. Second, the matter of mental illness was not initially raised. Gaining legitimacy would be difficult enough without compounding it by having to struggle with the stigma issue. The project was actually presented in its broader context of human services. Third, the organizer, in addition to obtaining names of persons to contact, was always careful to ask the respondent what he thought his reception would be by the suggested contact person. On several occasions, the organizer was advised not to contact Fr. X., a key clergy leader, until he had spoken with Frs. A., B., and C., and gained their support. He was also advised to begin his contact with a new individual with the information that he had been referred by so and so. These suggestions were carefully adhered to, and proved successful in reducing any potential opposition to the project, as well as in gaining legitimacy.

Several characteristics of the area became apparent from these initial interviews: The clergy enjoy a great deal of respect and deference; no single community-wide organization exists that represents the Southside as a whole; the community is self-contained and independent; the community is suspicious of outsiders wishing to help them, and especially suspicious of federal funds; and the community has tremendous strengths and resources, but is reluctant to admit that problems exist, particularly to "outsiders."

Many of those interviewed were cautious and questioned any project that seemed "parachuted" into the community by outsiders. One influential local priest remarked to the organizer after hearing a description of the proposed project, "Why are you picking on the Southside Poles?" Part of this came, we believe, from the strong stereotyping of the Polish ethnic community. There have been a number of incidents in the past where "missionaries" have gone into the Southside and attempted to "enlighten" the community. If we were going to succeed, our project had to overcome much of this hostility towards outsiders by the community leadership. Some of the positive factors that shape this community are pride, dignity, inner strength, and self-respect. The organizer staffing the project in Milwaukee was able to state honestly and without being patronizing that he had been brought up in a white ethnic neighborhood like the Southside, and therefore had some personal knowledge of the pride, values, and concerns of the white ethnic working class. His manner won him a degree of respect among these community leaders. If nothing else, it did convince them that the project was not a "missionary" endeavor to change or challenge the community. The leaders were assured that the community would have the final word on whatever transpired. It was also emphasized that we would be asking them neither for money nor large blocks of their personal time.

Although many community and institutional leaders were identified, they were not strongly tied with each other on an informal or formal basis. The Catholic parishes had selective, informal ties among various priests but actually were quite separate entities. There existed a series of ethnic, civic, social, and fraternal groups, of which the strongest and most respected included the Milwaukee Society of the Polish National Alliance, the Pulaski Council (an umbrella organization consisting of some 20 member groups), and Polanki (a women's cultural group). Neither block clubs nor action-issue groups were identified.

The worker maintained contact with approximately 15 people whom others had identified as key leaders of fraternal and civic groups, businessmen, clergy, and community institutions. It had become apparent that no single group, institution, or agency provided a central unifying focus for the Southside. The organizer spoke individually with the 15 "core" leaders about the possibility of forming a coalition to sponsor and direct the project. When most of these community figures seemed interested, he suggested that they meet with him, and the three authors of this book, to discuss particulars about the overall project.

In order that the reader may understand the flavor of the Southside community, brief sketches of a number of the core leaders are offered as a prelude to discussing our first "critical" meeting.

Fr. P., a diocesan priest in his 40s, was born and raised on the Southside. He has been a priest on the Southside for 20 years since his ordination. He is a traditional Polish priest, but he has recognized that the neighborhood has problems, and he was open to discussing mental health issues. Initially, Fr. P. was wary about the project. He was concerned that key project staff were of different ethnic backgrounds and were from different parts of the country than the Southsiders. He asked the organizer questions that implied, "Who are you? What do you want?" He said he had seen projects like this before, which came in with promises and left without doing anything. He had evidently been disappointed in the past and had a strong sense of pride. Once the project achieved legitimacy in Fr. P.'s eyes, he was very active. He served as the group's first President and was a most eloquent spokesperson. He dropped out of the project activities after several years because of his concern that the project was "spending too much money."

Fr. T., also a diocesan priest, is in his late 60s and was born and raised on the Southside. He has spent his entire career there. He loves his community very much, and knows it extremely well. Fr. T. is considered quite conservative, he is both respected and feared, and he has strong, outspoken opinions on a number of topics. He likes and supports SCO, but has at times suggested that the organization is too liberal and too humanistic. He gave SCO a multiroom office to use in one of his parish buildings, which served as the basis of its operations for three years. He supported SCO because he regarded its work as beneficial to his parishioners. It was Fr. T.'s intercession with a number of widowed parishioners that led to one of SCO's first self-help groups. His support of SCO was very important because of his great influence. When he began to support SCO, the respect and approval of other key Southsiders followed. His presence meant this was truly a neighborhood program and not merely some outside intervention.

Fr. J. is in his 40s and is an order priest from Chicago. He was new to the Southside, liberal, well educated with a degree in psychology, and served as pastor of an active, progressive parish. He feared that SCO would be too conservative, and was reluctant to get involved because conservative priests were involved. He sent another priest to represent him at the first SCO meeting. Then he came himself to the second meeting and told the other participants that he had not as yet made up his mind about joining SCO, that he just came to "check things out." The other group members urged him to join in and become part of the Board of SCO. Despite his concerns, he joined the Board and agreed to allow his name to be placed on the SCO stationery. This helped create a broadly representative group.

Sr. P., an order nun from Chicago in her 40s, was administrator of a Southside child welfare agency. She was wary of the project at first because she was new to the community and unsure if she should get involved. Initially very reserved, she soon became the President of the group. She carved out a key leadership role for women in the organization not traditional in this hierarchy.

Sr. M. is in her 60s and comes from Chicago. She held an administrative position at a Southside social service institution. Her order had abandoned habits, and this bothered a number of the Southside priests quite a bit. Initially she came because she was instructed to come and represent her agency at the meetings. She was very quiet at meetings. She proved to be an active member and a strong group participant once she became acclimated.

Mr. P. is a young (30s), very successful Polish-American lawyer with his own private practice. He was born on the Southside but now lives in the suburbs. He belongs to the Polish National Alliance (PNA) and has served as its president. He became involved with SCO at the behest of two other active PNA members. The PNA support of SCO was crucial in attracting strong, active community leadership like Mr. P. to SCO. He gradually became more and more involved with SCO because of his love for his old neighborhood. He was the first "lay" President of SCO. An extremely busy man, he dislikes many meetings, but provided strong, active leadership for SCO despite his limited available time.

Mr. S., in his late 60s, was born and raised on the Southside but now lives in the suburbs. He is a respected conservative Southside leader, serving as president of a local Polish Southside bank. His name came up over and over again in our exploratory meetings with Southside leaders, where he was considered a person we had to talk with. Initially suspicious about the project, he wanted to know more about our organizer. Eventually he became convinced the project would help the Southside and appointed Mr. N., the bank vice president, to represent him at the SCO meetings.

Mr. N., in his 60s, was born and raised on the Southside but now lives in the suburbs. He was vice president of the Polish bank and was given the assignment to come to SCO meetings. He participated actively with SCO and became its Treasurer.

Mr. R., in his 70s, was born and raised on the Southside. He was very active in the PNA and is a well known and established community leader. He seems to know everybody, and everybody seems to know him. His contacts and community reputation were invaluable to SCO's mission.

Fr. S., in his 70s, is director of the archdiocesan social service agency. He is a well respected archdiocesan priest holding a position of influence. He was not identified with the Southside, and had experience with the difficulties "outside" groups had in developing programs here. He was liberal but initially suspicious of SCO's efforts. Still, he was interested in having his agency serve effectively in the Southside.

As these descriptions show, many of the initial SCO members were well respected, older, established community leaders. Because they had initial doubts, the organization had to prove itself over time to be worthy of their respect and support. Their initial participation was principally due to the trust and confidence they placed in the Milwaukee field coordinator, though they remained very suspicious of this federally funded, Washington-controlled project. None of these individuals had ever worked together in a broad, neighborhood-based coalition such as SCO. They were curious. Would this idea work?

As a final step before the first meeting, the worker explained to each of the "core" leaders full details of the project, including the involvement of the National Institute of Mental Health and our view of the term *mental health*. He emphasized that the concept of mental health used in the project was not one of "locking up crazy people," but of encouraging the everyday expressions of respect, love, and unity that keep us all functioning in a healthy manner, both physically and mentally. It was explained that this concept recognized the crucial importance of cohesive and closely-knit communities, especially of the type often found in working-class ethnic areas such as the Southside. He underscored that the project would focus on preventing problems before they arose, rather than zeroing in on chronic problems or crisis situations. When the leaders voiced their approval of these concepts and their interest in proceeding with the project, it was time for the first organizational meeting.

Invitations to the initial meeting were sent to 17 leaders; 11 came. One of the area pastors was asked to host this first meeting and to act as temporary chairman. This pastor had a well deserved reputation for being more liberal than his fellow pastors on the Southside. Seven other priests were also invited, as were four civic leaders from the groups mentioned above. The administrators of a local day care center and hospital, both Felician nuns, were also invited because both these institutions, which were built through the nickel-and-dime contributions of Polish-Americans, were often cited as crucial to the community. Two other agencies were asked to send representatives: Catholic Social Services, which had established an outreach program two years earlier that was successfully operating through two of the Polish parishes, and an impressive senior citizen school located just north of the target area.

A number of the priests had some reservations about taking time away from their active schedules to attend the meeting. One pastor sent his assistant in his place. Five parish priests, one civic leader, and the administrators and staff of the four mentioned agencies were present. The chairman gave an excellent introductory talk, urging the gathering to unify and support the project. The key point made at the meeting was a description of the successful Catholic Social Services parish outreach project, concrete evidence of a successful small-scale mental health project on the Southside. Our project would strive to provide similar services with a wider and more diversified approach.

Certain activities, we said, were dictated by the grant from NIMH: A detailed needs study and assessment of resources had to be completed as the first step, and this would be followed by the creation of pilot projects that focused on the broad area of mental health. Beyond these two essentials, the newly formed coalition would guide the project and make all decisions as to its activities, including the selection of the projects. If the group did not feel this project was potentially beneficial to their community, then it would not be located there and a new field site would be sought. The choice was theirs, although we quivered at the possibility of a second defeat. The group cautiously accepted these terms. It agreed that such work was needed in their community. Interest was expressed in further details about project structure, and a second meeting was scheduled for the following month.

The next meeting was attended by 12 leaders. Each person was given a folder with descriptions, maps, and flowcharts that detailed the processes to be followed in the four-year program. After discussion, the leaders were asked if they wanted to go ahead. The answer was overwhelmingly positive. Entry had been achieved in a manner that empowered existing leadership rather than "parachuting" outside professionals.

In early 1977, the coalition chose a name—the South Community Organization (SCO)—and received donated office space in the rectory of a neighborhood church. Stationery was printed listing an expanded number of 18 members. Permanent officers were elected for the year. A target area of 22 census tracts was chosen.

The sponsoring coalition gave tremendous legitimacy to the project. Each person in the group represented a series of strong helping networks that were not necessarily closely linked with the others. The monthly meetings stimulated an exchange of information about these networks and generated ideas about the linking of resources. In earlier interviews, some of the leaders would say, "We do not have any problems in our community, and if we did, we would take care of them ourselves." Now they were talking about strengthening helping networks to meet the issues and concerns that traditional services could not always cope with. The process of determining needs and linking resources, which had begun at the first meeting of the group, continued in the ongoing dialogue.

Although the project had received initial endorsement and support, group members continued to suspect hidden elements in the agenda of the University of Southern California's Washington Public Affairs Center. There was also some fear that the grant's federal funding meant that the "Feds," not the Southsiders, would ultimately control what the project did. These feelings receded gradually as leaders developed more faith and confidence in the organizer and began to see that they really could control their activities themselves.

As demonstration programs developed over the course of the project, grassroots members were added to the Steering Committee of SCO. Over time, these people assumed much of the leadership and direction of SCO from the initial members. The founders still supported and helped the organization, but a number of them lacked the time necessary to develop and maintain the organization over a long period. Thus, after several years, leadership of SCO was a mixture of established community leadership and interested working people from the community who had not previously been identified as natural leaders. Once the South Community Organization attained legitimacy, the makeup of its membership gradually became similar to SECO's Neighborhood and Family Services Task Force in its representativeness.

The following few brief vignettes of SCO's new grassroots leaders will help to clarify who these individuals were and what they were like:

Mrs. J. is in her 40s, is married, and has three children. She became a member of the *Referral Directory* Committee. She is a nurse and was identified by community leaders as a "natural helper." She is active in the public schools—elementary and high school—and is very concerned about her neighborhood.

Mrs. C. is in her 30s, is a widow, and has two children. She was a member of SCO's Widowed Persons Group. Her first involvement with SCO was through her participation in a Family Communications Workshop. She dropped out before completing all of the workshop sessions. A follow-up phone call revealed that she felt the workshop did not address the special needs of widows. She was instrumental in helping SCO form its first support group for widows.

Mrs. P. is in her 50s, is married, and has three children. She is a native Southsider, is someone who knows everyone in her neighborhood, and is identified as a "natural helper." She works with many types of people, most extensively with teens, taking youth into her home on a temporary basis when they have no place to stay. She is active in the PNA Women's Auxiliary and church groups and is a key founding member of SCO's Family Communications Committee.

Mr. C. is in his 60s, is married, and has three children. He is an active community leader. He was retired from a career with the U.S. Postal Service and has spent most of his life on the Southside. Active in the church and local Democratic politics, Mr. C. is a natural helper who performs chore services and shops for his elderly neighbors. He was an active member of SCO's senior committee and later served as President of SCO.

FORMATION OF THE PROFESSIONAL ADVISORY COMMITTEE

A number of human service agency staff were among the 70 individuals contacted during the preliminary organizing efforts leading to the formation of the South Community Organization. Once SCO was formed, contacts began with other agencies. Soon some 50 agencies had been contacted. Many of these expressed interest in participating in the project and in becoming members of the Professional Advisory Committee (PAC).

Over 30 agencies were represented at the first PAC meeting in 1977. After a year of quarterly gatherings, meetings have been held since 1978 on a monthly basis. Agencies chose to participate in the project for different reasons. Some had experienced difficulty gaining entry, and therefore clients, on the Southside. Participation in this project seemed a way to gain a foothold on the Southside. Others joined to satisfy the demands of their funding agencies for community involvement, to develop relationships with other agencies, or simply to keep abreast of a new activity. The PAC worked actively with SCO committees as the project developed.

PAC members tended principally to be administrators and supervisors, although there were some line staff members. Membership often changed during the four years of the project. The descriptions of PAC members below are typical of the more active members.

Mr. D. is a young (30s) psychiatric social worker who was coordinator of a county mental clinic. He saw participation with SCO as a means for his agency to increase community contacts and make sure that their services were relevant to community needs. He was a very active member of the Family Communications Committee and participated as a group leader in a number of workshops.

Mrs. J., in her 40s, served with the Milwaukee County Mental Health Association and later with a private countywide family service agency. She had extensive experience with outreach programs and community-based programs. She was very eager to work with SCO and was a very helpful resource person. She helped train community facilitators for Family Communications Workshops. Later, as a staff member of the family counseling agency, she was an active team member of SCO's "wellness" project.

Mrs. L., head librarian of a neighborhood library, wanted to publicize library services—including workshops and informational programs. She wanted to attract more people to her branch, but was uncertain how to do it. She worked on PAC subcommittees, and her library hosted a "Family Fair" sponsored by SCO.

Joe K., director of a private, profit-making counseling service, wanted to make contact with other agencies—especially the nonprofit public agencies—and overcome prejudice he felt existed against his business. Outreach interested him and he evinced sincere interest in the provision of services to Southsiders. Eventually he set up a free self-help group for divorced men.

THE DATA-GATHERING PHASE

As in Baltimore, the early phase of the empowerment process included providing opportunities for neighborhood leaders to gather information about issues to be addressed and community assets. The staff was concerned that the community would view this research negatively and refuse to cooperate. SCO leaders, however, spread the word around the community that they were endorsing the research, that the findings would be used to help the community, and that it was okay to be interviewed. Refusal rates were very low.

SCO members analyzed census and other social indicator data, as well as interview data. The members demonstrated their "expert" knowledge of their community by explaining and elaborating upon formal statistics. For instance, census data indicated a high concentration of elderly, low-income, and foreign-born people in a certain neighborhood. A priest and a nun who were part of SCO and who were raised in that neighborhood explained that the statistics reflected the presence of many "displaced persons" from Poland who had settled there after World War II. Another member, who was himself a postwar immigrant, listed the various fraternal and veterans' organizations that these people belong to and provided the names of appropriate contact people. This example represents one important tenet of the project; that is, that residents are the "experts" on their neighborhood and that a truly accurate understanding of any community requires a combination of formal data and the informal knowledge of community residents.

The PAC was also actively involved in reviewing research findings. Two entire meetings were spent reviewing the findings. At the second meeting, a brainstorming session was held to discuss possible intervention strategies and projects that might stem from the data findings.

The research findings were similar to those in Baltimore; and while few new or shocking discoveries were made, the participation of local leaders and agency staff in the research process helped create a sense of energy and commitment for addressing unmet needs. Even more important, the issues defined as problems were chosen by SCO leaders, not by outside professionals. Among major findings: The term *mental health* was negatively "loaded"; people were often unaware of available agency services or were reluctant to use them because of mistrust or pride; Southsiders usually turned to community helpers—neighbors, friends, clergy—in times of need; the issues of poor family communications (especially between parents and teens) and the problems of single-parent families and the elderly were often cited.

The research process lasted seven months. Its duration created organizational problems for SCO. In a community organization, it is very hard to sustain interest, a sense of movement and action through a long study process. SCO members were anxious to launch pilot projects. They felt impeded by the extensive research and grant guidelines. Staff, in reaction, developed a more compact and easily implemented approach to assessing community needs, which was utilized in a later sister project.

Development of Demonstration Programs

The process of developing demonstration programs was much less time-consuming in Milwaukee than in Baltimore. SCO members gained the advantage of going through the process after Baltimore had already done it, learning from the Baltimore experience and adapting it to their own needs. Thus, since SCO liked Baltimore's guidelines for demonstration programs, they adopted them nearly *in toto*. SCO leaders were also more sophisticated and organizationally experienced than the Baltimore Task Force members, and thus could work faster. A corollary to this is the fact that SCO leaders were very busy and wanted to keep the planning meetings short and few in number. (On the other hand, in Baltimore, since meetings represented a support system for many Task Force members, the meetings became very significant as ends in themselves for many group members.)

After reviewing data findings and listening to suggestions from the PAC, SCO decided that its first priority was to help inform Southside residents of existing agency services. A one-page *Referral Directory* was developed that has since had three printings and has spun off a 60-page directory of services for senior citizens. Other projects included: a family communication workshop; support groups for divorced, widowed, and agoraphobics; a "wellness" project cosponsored by three private social service agencies and funded by the United Way; clergy agency luncheons; and a community helpers newsletter. Specific descriptions of some of these projects follow in chapter 11.

The Milwaukee experience demonstrates that the Baltimore findings were not idiosyncratic. Moreover, the presence of a medical college, with its high-technology models and a medical college department chairman, did not prevent successful neighborhood empowerment. The key features of the model, leaving key decisions about neighborhood needs to the neighborhood itself and creating links to skilled professional resources for illness, proved effective in practice.

CHAPTER 11

Advantages of a Neighborhood Support Systems Approach

In chapter 6, assumptions were listed related to: social class, ethnicity, and mental health; underserved and inadequately served population groups; community support systems; competency and power; and community and professional roles in mental health that undergird the Community Mental Health Empowerment Model. This chapter will consider the advantages of the neighborhood support systems approach utilized by the model within the general framework of those assumptions.

In the first part of this chapter, short vignettes of project experiences provide anecdotal evidence of the effectiveness of the model. These advantages are complementary and not mutually exclusive. A selected program may seem to highlight only one specific advantage; in reality, it may be seen to reflect numerous advantages. The second part of the chapter describes one specific demonstration project in detail, from planning through evaluation stages, to overcome this limiting process of "pigeon-holing." Our analysis shows how this single project exemplifies a number of advantages of the neighborhood system approach.

PROJECT VIGNETTES

1. *A Neighborhood Support Systems Approach can reach populations in need of assistance but unwilling or unable to seek professional help.*

• Through the action research process, it was determined that there were large numbers of ethnic, working-class women on the Southside of Milwaukee who were living alone. Many were divorced or widowed and considered at high risk for developing mental health problems. There is documented underutilization of mental health services by working-class women. They do not usually seek help from mental health centers or participate in organized self-help groups. This is a population that many mental health programs have difficulty reaching. As a result, it has remained largely underserved, except during psychiatric emergencies.

When this project began, there were no support groups for the divorced or widowed in the Southside target area. The data established that a need existed. We were not sure how to begin serving this population. Mental health professionals were eager to assist us, but we were concerned that a support group organized inside a mental health center would "label" participants as sick or crazy and would therefore not work. A group for young widowed persons with dependent children arose spontaneously when one woman initiated the idea with the project staff. Then a local pastor from the area approached our organizer and stated that he knew of a number of older widowed women in his parish who could also use a group. He gave the organizer several names. The widows were approached by the community organizer individually and were queried about their needs and interest in a support group. Each expressed reluctance or indifference. The organizer called the pastor and explained what had happened. The pastor said that he would contact the women himself. When the women found out that the pastor was supporting the program, they changed their minds and came to a meeting. Through interaction of staff and community, we developed two ongoing support groups for widows involving a total of over 50 women—one for older widows, the other for widows with children. Over time, staff involvement with both groups has decreased. The community organizers have gradually become consultants to the two groups as each has developed strong indigenous leadership.

Thus, as a result of efforts by networks of community clergy and neighborhood organizations, ethnic working-class women were drawn into self-help efforts sponsored under the aegis of the community. The organization of these groups reflects their own particular social and educational needs and interests. Initially, the widows were wary about involving professionals in their meetings. Over time, as group members developed rapport with one another and the groups coalesced, professionals were invited to speak and to serve as consultants on leadership development. In a reversal of what has been the "traditional" professional role, professionals served as advisors to the community-directed process. To be most effective for this population group, the initial organizing effort had to come from the community, not the professional sector.

• In Baltimore, a 72-year-old, mentally impaired gentleman was evicted from his apartment shortly before Thanksgiving Day for owing $200 in back rent. A young neighbor, knowing the man was too proud to ask agencies for assistance, called the Neighborhood Hotline for help (see the third vignette in category No. 3 for a detailed description of Hotline). He knew that Hotline was staffed by community volunteers in the neighborhood, many of whom had been helping people for years on their own before Hotline was formalized and its valuable assistance was organized. Hotline volunteers contacted agencies on behalf of the man, but immediate help was only sufficient to stay the eviction temporarily. There was no single agency that was willing or able to handle his problem satisfactorily from that point.

Hotline volunteers were distressed, knowing that by the time the necessary agency resources were mobilized, the man would be out on the street again. One Hotline volunteer became a special advocate for him. She called the landlord and strongly advised him that he was wrong in evicting the tenant. She pointed out to him a number of agencies he could have called for assistance. She complained that the tenant's worldly possessions were being put out on the street. The landlord replied that she shouldn't worry since he had few possessions anyway, and what he did have was not worth much. The community helper became incensed. She informed the landlord that what the man did have meant a great deal to him because they were his only possessions and he treasured them. The landlord took the tenant back in, and undoubtedly suffered from pangs of conscience on Thanksgiving. The community helper, in turn, agreed to continue to serve as advocate for the tenant by helping him obtain professional help. The gentleman was now willing to accept the professional assistance that he would not have initially accepted, since it was offered through the "legitimacy" of a community helper.

2. *A Neighborhood Support Systems Approach is built upon the strengths, not the weaknesses, of the community; it utilizes and enhances the neighborhood's preexisting systems of informal support, thus increasing the community's sense of competency and power.*

• On the Southside of Milwaukee, a federally funded community mental health center had for several years been aware of family communications problems in the neighborhood. Social workers from the center had broached the idea of communications seminars with the clergy as a means of addressing this issue. Failing to get an immediate favorable response, and aware of the fact that the Southside is a proud, tightly knit community that is unwilling to let a professional agency define its problems for it, the initial effort was abandoned. The mental health professionals had recognized and defined family communications as a problem, but the community and its leadership had not yet done so. As a result, the social workers from the mental health center could not gain access to the population, and their efforts ended in frustration.

SCO utilized a different approach to the same problem, this time with positive results. As stated in the description of the model and organizing strategies, community residents received assistance in developing a process to collect and analyze data on community strengths and needs. The emphasis in both cities, but especially in Milwaukee, was upon strengths and how those strengths could be utilized to address unmet community needs. Community residents and staff worked closely together to decide which people to talk to, what information to collect, and how to analyze the findings.

Once the data in Milwaukee was collected, a workshop to review the findings was held for community leaders and helpers. Many community helpers were surprised to find the extent to which family communications appeared to be a major problem. There was little reluctance to admit this, however, because they were interpreting and summarizing the results of raw data that they themselves had helped obtain from local community leaders and helpers. The definition of the problem clearly came from the community, not from "outside" professionals.

When the problem was recognized, people wanted to do something about it. A decision was made to employ the strength of existing neighborhood helpers. A committee of community helpers was organized, and "brainstorming" meetings were held with project staff to discuss possible interventions. The residents decided to ask agency professionals for their suggestions, inviting several professional representatives to the meetings. Once again, the professionals acted as advisors to the community-directed planning process.

The expanded committee decided to hold a four-part workshop on family communications. Community members took responsibility for getting people to the workshop by means of brochures, through bulletin announcements, and perhaps most importantly, through the informal communication channels of the community helpers. Professionals agreed to serve as staff coordinators at the workshop, following a plan devised by the entire committee. This first workshop was very successful; over 40 people participated, and a follow-up session was held for those who asked for more time to develop their communication skills. The first workshop led to a dozen more, with over 350 people participating. Over time, community helpers have taken on a larger role in staffing the workshops, including the teaching of communication skills.

● Another example of building upon strengths in the informal network was the formation of the On Our Own group in Milwaukee. After the first four-part family communications workshop, staff called residents who had attended only an initial session or two to find out why they had dropped out. One woman remarked that the sessions weren't relevant for her because she was a young widow with children—why didn't SCO offer something for widows? Staff replied that they would indeed like to develop activities for young widows like herself if there were sufficient interest.

Shortly afterward, project staff were speaking at a home-school meeting, discussing what SCO was doing in the community. After the meeting, a young widow approached the SCO staff and complained about a lack of support groups for young widows with dependent children. Now two residents were interested in a widows group. They were introduced to each other through the "brokerage" of project staff.

The two women, utilizing their own systems of informal support, contacted friends and neighbors, and SCO's first widows group was born—this one for young widowed persons with children. SCO staff played a much less prominent role in organizing this widows group than they did with the second one for older widows. The younger women were more responsive to the self-help notion. The knowledge of the two widow organizers about the problems of widowhood, and their contacts and relationships in the community, were also vital to the success of the effort.

● The organizational process of the project in Baltimore assisted community residents in developing the necessary competence and confidence to interact with professionals on a peer level. The description of clergy/agency/community activities in the second half of this chapter documents this in detail, but a short example here may also be helpful.

Although most Task Force members in Baltimore had considerable "experiential" knowledge of their community and its problems, they had little formal education. In early Task Force meetings, members would often defer to the "professional" knowledge of project staff members. The staff exercised restraint and restricted interventions to the limited areas in which their expertise could facilitate the process. At the same time, through training and technical assistance, the staff enhanced the capacity of Task Force members. Chapter 8 describes the involvement of Task Force members in the analysis of data findings. Through this process, residents gained factual and technical knowledge to add to their experiential knowledge. This made them more comfortable in interacting with agency professionals.

At a subsequent, combined Task Force–Professional Advisory Committee meeting, a discussion of intervention strategies ensued. Some recommendations were put forth by an agency professional. At this point, a Task Force member disagreed, and began flipping through her data book to cite research findings supporting her point of view. The agency professional became silent, not knowing how to respond. Other Task Force members became more vocal. Any remaining fears about interacting with professionals disappeared.

● In Baltimore, a number of natural helpers from the community had been involved for some time in visiting other local families that had suffered a recent death. A number of these helpers were themselves widows. Mrs. L., a 68-year-old widow, had lost her husband 13 years before. Knowing from personal experience the hurt and bewilderment of losing a loved one, she began on her own, comforting, supporting, and helping other people who were in mourning to adjust to death and continue their lives.

A local hospital involved with the project was concerned that supportive services be provided to families of deceased hospital patients, but their budget was limited and no new staff could be hired for this purpose. The SECO organizer, aware of the hospital's interest and the community helpers' experience, acted as a broker and brought the two groups together. The Peace at Sundown Program was thus formed. The neighborhood group recruited interested volunteers, and the hospital provided training, professional back-up, and referrals for the volunteers. The aim was to build and expand on what community helpers were already doing for the bereaved. The community quickly recruited 10 volunteers, but the hospital produced few referrals because of confidentiality problems involved in releasing the names and phone numbers of patients. The community helpers were undaunted; with back-up services and encouragement still available from professionals, they continued to locate their own referrals—from neighbors and friends as before, but now also through clergy, funeral directors, and obituary notices.

3. *A Neighborhood Support Systems Approach builds upon the unique ability of neighborhood residents to know what will work in their communities.*

● In Baltimore, a Community Health Education Network was formed through the project to promote positive mental and physical health. The Baltimore Field Coordinator said this of the rationale for the Network:

> Community residents felt that the agencies were concentrating their efforts only upon helping people after problems had already occurred. The residents believed that they themselves ought to take responsibility for prevention programs and activities. They felt comfortable in doing so, based upon their knowledge of the community and its helping networks.

The staff person's role with the mental health committee of the Network was to assist the committee in developing its ideas, but to do so while encouraging the residents' own initiative and common-sense approach to planning. The mental health committee of the Network decided to hold a four-part workshop on stress. The director of the Johns Hopkins University Hospital Community Psychiatry Program, a psychiatrist, agreed to run the workshop and to help plan the sessions with the community group. This planning process itself was a breakthrough for the community since there had been a considerable hiatus between 1971, when the Johns Hopkins psychiatrists left their very active community role, and the new linkage forged through this project.

The psychiatrist proposed to focus each workshop on one particular kind of stress (e.g., occupational, marital, or others). He wanted the entire four-part workshop preplanned with clear objectives. Community members wanted a looser, more flexible approach. After the discussion, the psychiatrist decided, in his words, to "wing it." He agreed to a planning meeting before each workshop session to review the last session and to plan the next.

At this point, the job of the social work staff was to help the committee plan for the workshop. The staff raised questions such as: How should the workshop be advertised? What will make people want to come? What will make people comfortable once they get there? Community residents supplied the answers. Community residents distributed flyers for the workshop, which were printed with little "bug" logos and said, "What's bugging you? Come to the Stress Workshop!" A potluck dinner was held before each session to make people more comfortable about attending. Social work staff, coming from a much different frame of reference, felt that they could never have come up with these "angles." The residents were correct in their approach on how to get people to come. The series was very successful, with up to 70 persons attending individual sessions. A tremendous rainstorm struck the community one hour before the final session, flooding the streets and disrupting traffic. The planning committee was all set to cancel that last session when people began arriving, by foot, with umbrellas and without! Attendance was as high as it had been at other sessions. Responses on a written evaluation form circulated at the last session were extremely favorable.

A number of residents who attended the workshop have subsequently told planning committee members that they now feel it's safe to talk about stress and problems, and commented that "the shrink was okay," or "psychiatrists aren't bad." This response was remarkable, coming from a community where going to a psychiatrist for help carries with it a significant stigma. Many residents who would not ordinarily have attended such a workshop participated because of its community sponsorship, informal setting, extensive publicity, and the personal contact and trust they had with planning committee members. The roles of project staff and community residents were symbiotic. The staff knew what decisions and steps had to be made in organizing a workshop, the community residents knew what would or would not work in their community. Several times in this planning process, staff had to "bite the bullet" and refrain from interfering with residents' ideas of how they wanted to proceed.

● In Milwaukee, data findings from the project showed that many community residents did not know where to go for help. A committee of residents and agency professionals, which was formed to discuss this problem, quickly agreed that a referral directory for use by community residents was needed. Considerable disagreement, however, arose over what form this directory should take.

Agency professionals favored a comprehensive directory for Southsiders with a complete listing and program description of all agencies serving the area. It would be a smaller version, about 20 pages, of the *Directory of Agencies* published in Milwaukee by United Way. The community residents listened, then responded: "That sounds interesting—but Southsiders won't use it." They then suggested a one-page *Directory* with listings by problem or population group (alcoholism, problems of the elderly, health care, emotional distress, etc.). They felt it should contain only the most essential services. The professionals were concerned about leaving some agencies out. They did not want to be accused by other professionals of being biased or unfair. In the end, the professionals acceded to the wishes of the community residents. A two-sided, one-page *Directory* listing 45 agencies in 17 service categories was developed. It was printed on heavy folded stock to be posted near the telephone (another suggestion of residents). Printing costs were covered through grants from several Milwaukee foundations. The *Directory*, now in its third edition, has been widely distributed—over 30,000 copies—through churches, neighborhood stores, community groups, ethnic clubs, and agencies. Specific directories for elderly and youth services have also been developed as a result of this small initial effort.

The principle of working through informal systems of support and relying, then building, on the capacity of local residents to know what works in their community sounds like a simple enough principle to follow. In practice, this may not be the case, as the following vignette illustrates.

● In Baltimore, through the efforts of the project, a Hotline run by neighborhood residents was established to help institutionalize the natural work of neighborhood helpers. Because Hotline is staffed by natural helpers and not professionals, it reaches some individuals who would not ordinarily seek professional help. The idea for this Hotline came from Mrs. H., 65, a long-time resident of South East Baltimore and a natural helper who has been advising people from her kitchen for years. The role of the project coordinator in Baltimore was to help Mrs. H. and other interested residents get the Hotline off the ground. According to the staff member, "Mrs. H. and the other residents knew what they wanted to do and how they wanted to do it. I helped them be aware of all the steps and decisions that had to be made before the Hotline became operational." As the planning proceeded, the project staff became uncomfortable with its methods. Since Hotline was part of a research and demonstration project, good records of each call and of the follow-up action seemed important. The residents weren't particularly interested in this. They felt that written records were unimportant. Staff soon realized, however, that Hotline volunteers, many of whom had been helping people in their community on their own for years, did indeed have their own system of accountability. After a volunteer aided a caller, if she could get his/her phone number, she would call back and see if the person obtained the help needed. Volunteers were already doing follow-up; they simply were not recording it precisely the way project social workers expected to have it done. We realized that we were asking Hotline to run as if it were a professionally staffed operation. We had expected the residents to adapt to our structure, not create and maintain their own. This violated every principle we thought we were following on this innovative project. Once we recognized this, we let the residents operate Hotline their way. We tried to document Hotline's successes and failures anecdotally, through individual, personal contacts between staff and volunteers and by group meetings with Hotline volunteers.

4. *A Neighborhood Support Systems Approach can enhance consumer involvement in service delivery and make agencies accountable on the neighborhood level.*

• In Baltimore, a dozen elderly residents frantically came to the front door of a community helper well known for her advocacy skills. They were very concerned that their Social Security checks had not arrived that morning. They did not know what to do and were very frightened. The Social Security check is their only income. They pleaded with the neighborhood helper to "call somebody up and do something." The neighborhood helper, aged 65 and also dependent on her Social Security check, was also nervous but hid her anxiety from the group. She called the local Post Office and complained. She was told that the mailman had left early in the morning with the Social Security checks. Since it was already 2:00 p.m. when she called, she pressured the Post Office to track down the lost mailman. At this point she explained the situation to her elderly neighbors and urged them to go back to their houses and wait. They refused and stayed on her doorstep. A short while later, the mailman arrived, having been roused from a local drinking establishment to find an angry group of Social Security recipients shouting out their names and demanding their checks. For the mailman, it was an experience in accountability he will never forget.

• In Milwaukee, the unmet needs of the aged were a major concern uncovered by our research. A Task Force of the aged, called the Senior Task Force, was formed. Through the assistance of the University of Southern California, Washington Public Affairs Center, they received subcontract funds on a three-year model project funded by the Administration on Aging. The grant was aimed at strengthening neighborhood-based support systems for the elderly in a manner very similar to that of the NIMH grant of the Neighborhood and Family Services Project.

The Task Force felt that the aged on the Southside needed more opportunities for socialization. When they found out that Milwaukee County was planning to build a senior center on the Southside, they urged a county planning committee to expand the center to include facilities for an "eating together" program. Soon after the planning committee gave approval, the board of supervisors announced that not only would the center not be expanded, but it would not be built at all because of budgeting problems. The senior citizens became incensed. A petition was circulated in support of building an expanded senior center with a meal site in it. About 3,000 signatures were collected. A group of 40 to 50 elderly people from the Southside came to a board of supervisors meeting to present their petitions and to urge the supervisors to build the needed facility. Seldom having experienced pressure like this from the Southside, the supervisors were impressed. They agreed to build a senior center with an eating facility. The community won.

Both the supervisors and community residents learned a lesson in accountability from this experience. Supervisors used to making decisions about the Southside with little consultation with the community realized that they must now operate differently. Residents, previously apprehensive about confronting high officials, now feel strong and proud about having asserted their interests. This feeling of empowerment has spread to other matters. The seniors now feel more confident that they can in fact have some say over decisions affecting their lives.

5. *Creating linkages between Neighborhood Support Systems and mental health and human service programs can reduce fragmentation of services, provide help in a more effective manner, and "demystify" the role of professionals.*

• In Baltimore, a low-income elderly man in poor health and on crutches was caring for his invalid wife at home. He could not bear to send her to a nursing home, so he began selling their lifelong household belongings in order to afford care for her at home. Medical insurance would cover the cost of "institutional" care for the woman in a nursing home, but would not cover home care. When his wife died, social workers from the local health department wanted the man removed to a nursing home because he required too much assistance to live alone. The NFSP worker discussed the reaction of the man and his neighbors to this suggestion: "He was still grieving for his lost wife when the agency worker told him that he would have to leave his home. He had lived in the same neighborhood for most of his life and just couldn't bear to leave. The social worker was suggesting what she thought was best for her client, but his neighbors had other ideas." Through the Neighborhood and Family Services Project Hotline, a community helper learned of the matter. She contacted neighbors and mobilized a coordinated, accountable, unfragmented rotation system of community helpers to aid him. As a result, he still lives in his own home, with neighbors providing the necessary grocery shopping, cooking, cleaning, and household maintenance that enable him to stay in the community.

Professional services now serve as back-up for the efforts of these community helpers.

The role of the project staff in this situation was coordinative. Community residents came up with their own plan to help this man, and project staff helped them to communicate and coordinate their efforts. In so doing, they helped educate agency professionals in the workings of neighborhood networks.

Another short vignette describes how Hotline creates linkages between community and professional helpers.

● One day a man called Hotline and said that he was going to kill himself. The Hotline volunteer did everything she could do to keep him talking. After a few minutes, she asked him if he had dressed. When he said no, she told him to get dressed right away and she would call him back in 5 minutes. In those 5 minutes she called the Crisis Clinic at Baltimore City Hospital and arranged for a trained professional to go to the man's house and take him to a local psychiatric hospital for immediate help. The Hotline volunteer was quick, perceptive, competent, and effective because she knew all the resources in the community, and she was personally acquainted with professionals at the Crisis Clinic. She called them directly and requested their assistance. When dealing with large bureaucracies like hospitals, this feat is not easy. The process described above can work only if lay helpers and mental health professionals learn to work in tandem to assist neighborhood people in times of crisis. In this situation, the expertise of the lay helper, coupled with the resources and accessibility of the community Hotline and agency professionals, may have prevented a suicide.

● In Milwaukee, the organization of a Professional Advisory Committee of agencies serving the Southside substantially reduced the fragmentation of services. Representatives of some 30 agencies met on a regular basis over a three-year period to discuss ways to coordinate their efforts, thus simplifying the process of seeking and receiving help for Southside residents. This was the first organized, ongoing group of Southside agencies in a decade or more. Initial efforts focused on information-sharing among agency representatives. A looseleaf *Directory of Southside Agency Services*, featuring one-page descriptions of each agency's programs and services, was developed for use by agency staff. It provided much greater detail than the "red book" of community agencies for the entire metropolitan area. Other specialty directories, such as one on alcohol and drug abuse, followed. Many agency representatives have found these directories invaluable for aiding multi-problem clients requiring the services of several agencies.

Another effort of the PAC was a four-day Southside Spring Fair with workshops for children, teens, adults, and the elderly. Brochures on individual Southside agencies, as well as copies of a *Central Agency Directory*, were circulated. Several hundred persons attended. Community residents and agency representatives were pleased with results. An indirectly anticipated byproduct of the Advisory Committee was the fostering of informal relationships and linkages among service providers, which resulted in an increase of beneficial referrals.

The success of the PAC of Southside agencies led to similar spin-off groups of agencies focusing on particular population groups. The Southside Youth Committee and a half dozen youth, for example, assisted representatives of almost every agency working with Southside youth. They shared information on problems and sponsored two successful teen workshops, the first for teens and their parents, the second for teens only. Over 30 persons attended each workshop. Evaluations were very positive. A teen rap group was formed because teens asked for an ongoing support mechanism. The Committee and the PAC also published a *Directory of Southside Youth Services*.

● In Baltimore, a clergy/agency/community seminar attracted over 80 persons. A detailed analysis of this seminar is offered in the second half of this chapter. Small mixed groups of clergy, agency, and community helpers met to explore their strengths and resources during part of the seminar. At a debriefing meeting, a clergyman remarked that the community helpers from his parish learned for the first time that professionals didn't "have all the answers." In previous dealings with professionals, these community helpers had felt "one down." Now they felt encouraged, more confident about their ability to go out and really help people. At the seminar, they had equal participatory status with professionals; this enabled them to penetrate the "mystique" of professionalism.

A PROGRAM IN DETAIL—LINKING CLERGY, COMMUNITY, AND PROFESSIONAL HELPING NETWORKS[1]

Late in the autumn of 1977, a young Lutheran minister from South East Baltimore proposed to the SECO Task Force staff coordinator that

[1]A fuller version of this program appears in D. Biegel & A. Naparstek "The Neighborhood and Family Services Project: An Empowerment Model Linking Clergy, Agency Professionals, and Community Residents." In A. Jeger & R. Slotnik (Eds.), *Community Mental Health and Behavioral-Ecology: A Handbook of Theory, Research, and Practice*. New York: Plenum Press, 1982.

a seminar be organized to bring clergy and agency staff together. New to the community and unaware of its resources, he felt that he and other clergy could learn much from a workshop with agencies. Project data indicated that lay and professional helping networks were fragmented. The project coordinator enthusiastically referred the minister to *both* the Task Force and Professional Advisory Committee, a crucial step because community representatives, not the staff, had jurisdiction over all major project decisions. Both the Task Force and the PAC responded positively.

A Task Force committee of clergy, human service agency staff, and community residents was formed. Clergy in South East Baltimore, from staff experience, had busy schedules and were reluctant to attend meetings. The number and length of planning meetings needed to be strictly limited: Only two planning meetings would be held, and each meeting would run only 90 minutes.

Twelve persons were recruited for the committee—six clergy (four Catholic and two Protestant) five agency professionals, and one Task Force representative. The committee was staffed by two persons. Committee members were selected on the basis of interest in the seminar, willingness to commit time to planning, and a positive reputation among their respective colleagues.

Project staff developed some planning strategies prior to the first meeting. Staff contacted a wide range of clergy before the first meeting of the committee to gauge interest in a seminar. Agency staff were expected to attend the seminar willingly since such activities are a normal professional staff commitment. Clergy might be harder to reach. We were pleasantly surprised to find unanimous interest among the 20 clergy we spoke to—evidence, we believed, of a strong unmet need.

Staff suggested to the committee that the seminar be cosponsored by as many different clergy and agency groups as possible, helping to ensure widespread "ownership" and helping to attract participants. This tactic proved a key factor in the seminar's success.

Three full planning committee sessions and one subcommittee meeting took place over four months before the actual event in April, 1978. Attendance was excellent; no meeting had fewer than 10 persons present.

The first planning meeting resembled a seminar in miniature. Some clergy were meeting colleagues for the first time. Some agency professionals and clergy were interacting for the first time as well (the agency professionals present already knew each other). Catholics and Protestants became acquainted; so did clergy of the same denomination. Two young Protestant ministers who had never met, but who had

similar interests, were especially pleased to meet. The kinds of relationships and linkages we hoped the seminar would encourage began
to form in the planning stages.

The focus and purpose of the seminar preoccupied the first two
planning sessions. At first, the committee favored an agenda with skills
training and discussion of specific problems. This approach was determined to be too ambitious for a first seminar. Gradually the focus of the
seminar shifted to clergy and agency professionals getting to know one
another—and the ways they could work together to help people in
need. Staff's "hidden agenda" was for the seminar to be the first of an
ongoing series. The committee members themselves articulated this as
a goal early in the planning process, without hints or pressure from the
staff. Numerous topics could not be covered in one seminar. For ongoing linkages to be established successfully between clergy and human
service agencies, it became evident that a series of seminars or other
activities were required.

The planning process also revealed that there were many "natural
helpers" in the community—friends, neighbors, co-workers, barten-
ders, and so forth—who helped persons in need (in fact, many of these
natural helpers were interviewed in the research phase of the project).
Late in the planning process, the scope of the seminar was enlarged to
include clergy, agency, and community helpers.

The committee agreed to the staff's recommendations for cosponsorship by 10 clergy and agency organizations. Three separate mailings
were sent to prospective seminar participants, including all clergy in
South East Baltimore, all Professional Advisory Committee agencies,
additional selected South East Human Service Agency Staff, and
selected guests. Personal contact was made by Task Force representatives to interest community helpers.

Participants were asked to preregister two weeks before the date
of the seminar. By the preregistration deadline, only 15 responses had
been received, only one from a clergyman! One week before the seminar, only 25 persons had preregistered. Staff began to worry that the
seminar would be a failure. When the final planning committee meeting was held, committee members took full responsibility for personal
recruiting efforts to increase preregistrations. Their efforts proved successful; by the day of the seminar, over 60 persons were preregistered.

It was evident by this last meeting that committee members had
taken "ownership" of the seminar. Decisions on steps that needed to be
taken to increase the registration and the division of responsibilities for
tasks needing accomplishment were quickly decided on by committee
members with minimal staff input. A healthy tension developed

between the Catholics and Protestants, and between clergy and agency professionals, each wanting to avoid the embarrassment of a low turnout by their respective members. Ultimately 85 persons attended—32 clergy, 35 agency staff (representing 23 agencies), 15 community helpers, and 3 project staff. It was the largest turnout of clergy anyone could recall for any single event in South East Baltimore. The day lasted from 8:30 A.M. to 3:00 P.M., mostly occupied in small group meetings. In the morning, after some welcoming remarks, a short skit entitled "Family on the Rocks" portrayed a family with multiple problems. Seminar participants broke into small, unmixed groups of clergy, agency, and community residents. Each group was charged to focus on the roles that its members could play in helping the family and to discuss ways in which their group could work together more effectively to help the family address its problems. In a second small group breakdown, each group consisted of clergy, agency, and community representatives mixed together. Their focus was on ways that the three groups—clergy, agency, and community helpers—could work together better to help those with problems. Emphasis was placed on an examination of the strengths and weaknesses of each helping group.

In a general session before lunch, each group shared the high points of its discussion with the rest of the seminar. After lunch, a guest speaker detailed important contributions that the clergy and agency each could make in the helping process. The day ended with a general discussion of "Where Do We Go From Here?"

A sense of excitement seemed to fill the seminar room throughout the day. This was confirmed by written evaluations at the end of the day. Out of 42 participants responding 95% rated the seminar as "good" or "excellent," and 98% of the participants stated that they would like to be involved again in similar future activities. Almost half of the participants responding to the written evaluation form, 20 individuals, volunteered to work on a committee to help plan possible future activities. Groundwork was laid for continued community–professional interaction.

Participants at the seminar succeeded in developing initial linkages with each other. In comments at the end of the day, one nun, a parish school principal, said she came to the conference wanting to get help for two of her students. She came away from the seminar with the names and phone numbers of two specific agency helpers. She was very pleased.

The seminar seemed to create increased respect and understanding by helper groups of the role of other helping groups. For example, a number of clergy remarked how surprised and pleased they were that so many community helpers appeared able to reach individuals who wouldn't go to agencies for help. Similarly, a number of professionals who believed that professional "credentials" were essential to help people in need, went home with healthy questions about that belief.

As promised at the April seminar, in order to facilitate informal linkages, all participants were sent a list of names, phone numbers, and affiliations of seminar attendees, as well as written suggestions from the participants for possible future activities. An enlarged Planning Committee soon met to review the evaluation and feedback concerning the April seminar and to plan future activities.

In reviewing ideas for the future, there were many suggestions for follow-up. A number of seminar participants suggested a future half-day seminar to be held on a quarterly basis. The Planning Committee accepted this idea. Additional activities were also planned so that there would be more frequent interaction among the clergy, agency, and community helpers.

Melding the ideas of two committee members, monthly Case Study/Brown Bag Lunches were organized to combine informal get-togethers and activities with a substantive focus. The committee decided to adopt the Lancaster Case Study Method, developed by the Lancaster Theological Seminary, for use with an interdisciplinary group of helpers. The objective of the Lancaster approach is to develop and perfect a method of exchange among clergy around case material which will aid them in a responsible understanding of the events and decisions that must be made arising out of them.

The Brown Bag Lunches were scheduled on a monthly basis from 11:00 A.M. to 1:00 P.M. and were open to clergy, agency, and community helpers. Participants were divided into mixed groups (clergy, agency, and community helpers) of about eight persons each, with each group considering a different case. The cases were written and presented by a clergy, agency, or community helper, with one-case presentation being made per group. Each case was written in advance by the presenter according to an outline given to them. Staff assisted community helpers in preparing their outlines. Prior to the start of the group discussion, the moderator described the process to be followed, the roles of Presenter and Group Leader, and the time sequence (the Lancaster design was slightly modified to meet the project's purposes). The moderator emphasized that participants were not there to judge the "competence" of the presenters, but rather to seek alternative ways to help solve problems and needs as indicated in the cases, to utilize the various kinds of expertise represented in each group, to consider workable solutions based on the specific information in the cases, and to explore the various community resources in South East Baltimore available to help with the case problem.

Monthly seminars have been held and attended by approximately 25 to 50 persons per session ever since. Feedback from participants after each session has been very positive, as has been the staff analysis of what took place at these sessions. The case study luncheons have achieved a number of goals directly related to the advantages of the neighborhood Support Systems Approach that we outlined in the first part of this chapter.

Through these seminars, professionals have become aware that many persons unwilling to go to them for help do receive assistance from clergy and community helpers. Agency professionals have been sensitized to the issue of stigma in use of services, and have begun to realize that certain client groups may be best reached by professionals working through the informal support systems in the community. Professionals have also come to understand, appreciate, and value the "experiential" knowledge of lay helpers and their unique abilities to know what will work in their communities. Before the sessions began, many professionals doubted that community helpers had anything to offer them. Over time, however, through seeing these helpers both describe their own roles in helping people and make suggestions concerning how the professionals could become more effective, the opinions of the professionals reflected growing respect for the competence of these untrained, often uneducated helpers. In fact, a holistic, comprehensive approach to problem solving has been developed by group participants, and there has been a growing acceptance of the need for ongoing linkages among all helpers, lay and professional, to address the issue of fragmentation of services.

Fragmentation of services has also been addressed in other ways through these sessions. Knowledge of new and/or additional community resources in South East Baltimore to meet identified needs was acquired by group participants. The sheer number of helping resources makes it difficult even for experienced helpers to know precisely where to refer people in need. The sessions have also helped to integrate new helpers into the community. Since churches and human service agencies experience high staff turnover rates, these sessions have helped introduce new helpers to the community and its resources.

The feedback that lay helpers have received from their helping peers has reinforced their sense of competency and power. For example, a young clergyman remarked that in his work he received feedback from many sources pertaining to the performance of his clerical duties—except in the area of counseling parishioners. The feedback he received from the case study sessions on his counseling abilities was invaluable to him because he really had no way to judge whether or not he was performing his helping role adequately. Neighborhood helpers are often in the same isolated position in regard to feedback. Many of them have also remarked how these sessions have aided them. The reinforcement and validation by professionals of the performance of lay helpers enabled them to feel that they have the ability and expertise to interact with professionals on a peer level. They found out that they often have as many "answers" as the professionals do. For some, this was a startling discovery.

The sessions have indicated areas of unmet need within the community and have stimulated the development of new services and approaches to meeting those needs. It became evident through a number of case study examples that youth problems were increasing, and helpers were frustrated, not knowing exactly how to respond. An all-day seminar was planned to focus on this issue, and over 80 helpers attended. Participants rated this seminar highly and formed a committee to develop intervention suggestions arising from the day.

Finally, the sessions have protected helpers against "burnout" by providing time to ventilate, share frustrations and problems, and develop expanded informal systems of social support. Many professional and community helpers now interact on a first-name basis. A clergyman wishing to refer his client to the Johns Hopkins Community Psychiatry Program can now call Art, a psychiatrist he knows, or Fred, a social worker, whom he personally has confidence in. Professionals in turn are relying more on the clergy, not merely as a source of financial support for their clients, as was often the case, but as associates and colleagues.

CHAPTER 12

Issues and Limitations

The Community Empowerment Model is not a panacea for the community mental health movement or a blueprint that all other communities ought to follow step-by-step. This was a useful, successful experience, but a model cannot serve as all things to all people. The critical reader will by now recognize that there are inherent limitations in this model as in others. Moreover, these are difficult issues that must be addressed in any effort to adopt the model to other neighborhoods. Some of these concerns have been raised at conference presentations of the project. Agency professionals have posed others, and project staff have also cited issues that need to be dealt with in efforts to adopt these ideas and examples elsewhere. This chapter addresses the chief issues and limitations identified in the practical implementation and testing of the model, as well as our consideration of the limits of the conceptual framework.

Over the past two decades there has been a pattern of looking for "quick, one-stop" fixes. The concerns have been of such intensity that valid partial solutions have at times been pounced on as "the answer." Then it became all too easy in the ambience of the eighties to discard such programs as worthless. Each approach tends to go through a biphasic curve of uncritical enthusiasm followed by uncritical rejection. This chapter is included to temper and dampen these plans. With a more critical introduction, perhaps models can be spared the hypercritical "assassination" phase.

1. Community organizations, due in large part to their newness, their frequently unstable funding bases, and their operation as "advocacy" groups responding to issues as they arise, often cannot engage in long-range planning or even ensure a stable continuity of operation in the short run. How then can professionals be expected to form partnerships with such organizations?

171

Community organizations, by definition, must be fluid, changing entities. A representative neighborhood entity will reflect the needs, the networks, and the current leadership of neighborhoods. In contrast, high-technology health institutions, like hospitals, are built around a consensus of concepts, a scientific base that changes slowly. The process-oriented institution and objective-oriented institution are very different. Fluidity and change need not necessarily be obstacles preventing work with community organizations, but the nature of the neighborhood groups must be fully understood by professionals. Moreover, high-technology care for the very ill must be rendered in stable institutions. This is why the public hospital, open to constant winds of political change, has tended to be a failed institution. Similarly, the community mental health center, which sought to couple high-technology medical care and true neighborhood impact, had difficulty accomplishing either mission. Polarization tended to occur. Only charismatic leadership embodying both tasks enhanced by spectacular Board construction brought full success.

The fluidity of community organizations caused numerous challenges in the project. For example, in Baltimore, there were "ups and downs" and many changes of personnel and leadership at SECO. During the four years of the project, SECO had three different executive directors and other internal staff changes. These changes required adaptation by the project staff around such issues as project goals, objectives, and budget. Yet because of the preparedness to deal with process issues as they came up, the changes did not adversely affect the outcome of the project. The staff had worked for and with community organizations before, knew what to expect, and were prepared to deal with change. This fluidity, in our view, is a sign of meaningful community process. Projects that are as unchanging as an old type health institution probably have not developed true neighborhood roots. Health professionals must be cautious not to demand "clones" of their own institutions as a condition of neighborhood linkage.

2. Most community organizations are "advocacy" groups. Advocacy groups often make enemies in the community. How can these organizations be expected to develop partnerships with as broad an array of community and professional groups as is required by this model?

This issue must be carefully considered in selecting a community organization as a local project sponsor. Community organizations seeking to enhance the power of neighborhood residents often use confrontation as an organizing tactic. While this can be both advantageous and necessary in meeting a group's goals, segments of the community necessary for successful partnerships may be alienated by such tactics. Our experience is that, while certain community organizations might be seen so negatively as to preclude the formation of the partnerships, this has proven the exception rather than the rule. Most groups are likely to be viewed positively by some people, negatively by others. The health organization *linked* to advocacy groups need not accept responsibility for specific advocacy enterprises any more than the neighborhood accepts responsibility for medical decisions. Developing clear boundaries is essential to such linkages.

In Baltimore, some health professionals were suspicious of SECO because of its past history of confrontation organizing. There was also considerable respect for what the organization had accomplished. In addition, project staff made clear to agency professionals that, though the Neighborhood and Family Services Project was part of SECO, the tactics and methods were those of network building. One cannot expect fundamentally conservative, older institutions and agencies to become part of a confrontation/advocacy system. The fact that SECO had a community development arm whose philosophy was partnerships, and that this arm had a very good record of success, lent credence to our assertion.

3. Mental health does not seem to be a sufficiently "vivid" or "exciting" issue to serve as the basis for community organization. Housing, education, zoning, sanitation, and so forth, all seem to be more pressing immediate concerns on the neighborhood level. Will community organizations be interested enough in mental health? Can "issue" organizing and "human service" organizing both operate out of one community organization?

From the beginning, this project faced challenges based on this issue. Mental health is realistically *not* a high-priority community issue. Indeed, the placement of a mental health project in a grassroots community organization can lead to organizing difficulties.

This is exactly why neighborhood approaches are needed. One cannot expect the problem to disappear just because a project is announced. These are long, hard process issues. When project staff initially began organizing the Task Force, prospective members would agree to come to a meeting, but would often cancel at the last minute because of what they regarded as higher priorities—attending a zoning hearing, for example. There seemed to be no sense of immediacy; mental health problems and issues could be discussed at any time; but a

zoning hearing needed to be attended that day. Community organization issues do have immediacy; they are by definition action-oriented
and are often scheduled on short notice to respond to a crisis. Human
service meetings may deal with important problems and issues, but
they tend to be oriented to planning, not action; planning meetings do
not *have* to happen at a specific time. But once members became
invested in the Task Force and its projects, their priorities *changed*.
People became very committed to the Task Force and its agenda. When
this happened, the meetings began taking priority over other commit-
ments. When mental health leaves the levels of slogans and when real
people with real issues are involved, saliency is achieved.

In reality, we were not simply organizing people around mental
health, but around the concept that neighborhoods contain within them
many strengths and resources to help people in need, and that neither
professionals nor community members themselves were fully aware of
these strengths. Residents became excited as they identified these
strengths and recognized how they could be used. Empowerment was
actually the independent variable, mental health the dependent. The
community empowerment philosophy, of course, meshes well with the
ideological basis of most community organizations.

Most community organizations initially coalesce and grow strong
around "issues." As they mature, many become involved in economic
development and human service delivery. SECO in Baltimore followed
this route; the project at SECO increasingly became part of the group's
total human services network. SCO in Milwaukee did develop around
human service issues and has developed successfully.

Organizing around issues *and* for human service within one organization requires that both staff and residents become fully aware of
variances between different organizing strategies. Mental health needs
and prevention are not popular, immediate "gut" issues. They do raise
fears and concerns. Some residents had doubts about participating in
self-help groups and workshops, feeling that this implied they were
weak or lacked pride and independence. Some were apprehensive
because they felt they might be required to reveal "family secrets."
Others felt intimidated by professionals, or felt that all planning should
be left to "the experts." People on planning committees and the Board
needed to learn that the experts didn't have all the answers, and that
no one knows a community and its needs better than the people who
live in it. Unlike classical organizing, which is characterized by clear-
cut victories (such as getting an abandoned house razed), preventative
mental health projects do not yield definitive or immediately visible
results that can be celebrated. When dramatic breakthroughs do occur

in a self-help group or workshop, they can be appreciated by the participants, but usually pass unnoticed by the larger community. They do not represent a highly visible victory such as obtaining a traffic light at a dangerous street corner. In human service organizing, self-growth of community residents is an important and explicit goal. In issue organizing, self-growth of residents may also be important, but it tends to be a by-product of achieving action goals.

4. The project seems to require exceptional staff who have a combination of clinical, group work, and community organization skills. Aren't such practitioners hard to find?

This is an age of specialization. Individuals with all of the attributes needed for an endeavor such as this one are hard to come by; in-service training is therefore vital. Although this project did not include a formalized in-service training program, staff worked as a team and learned from each other, realizing that particular staff members had areas of exceptional expertise. Administrative staff spent significant amounts of time training new staff members through supervision and by accompanying them to community meetings.

Based on our experience with the project, the concept of the role of the staff needs to be expounded. Field staff played a critical role in helping to organize community residents and in keeping them involved throughout the course of the project. Because of the nature of human service organizing, a combination of organizational and clinical talents are required in staff. The organizer must have a multidisciplinary approach to community work. He/she needs a strong background in classical community organizing, that is, a knowledge of the process of community self-actualization; also necessary are professional human service skills in facilitating the growth and development of individuals and groups; and, finally, political skills are basic for the survival and success of any community worker.

A basic assumption of human service organizing is that neighborhood residents, by virtue of their own life experiences living in the neighborhood, have the experiential knowledge necessary to develop programs designed to meet the human service needs of their community. Not all residents, however, have the skills and self-confidence necessary to accomplish this. It is the organizer's responsibility to facilitate residents' growth through the development of skills and self-confidence. The most important function of the organizer is a supportive one, the "Go ahead, I'm right behind you" philosophy, which encourages residents towards achievements they may never have thought possible. This function of the organizer differs significantly from classical organizing in that there is a much greater emphasis on facilitating the growth of individuals: In classical organizing there is less direct attention to dealing with personal issues.

A fundamental aspect of human service organizing is the organizer's ability and responsibility to help residents articulate their philosophy through a group process. This was accomplished in our project initially through drawing up on criteria or guidelines for programs, and then was continued through committee work in the program development process.

Essential to human service organizing is the need for the organizer to work with individual residents, not as sick people, poor people, or clients, but as equal partners in a network-building process. Clinicians are advised to keep a "professional distance" and remain in role, but the organizer needs to demystify his professional identity. He/she must not hide behind degrees, jargon, or other professional traits that tend to separate the organizer from neighborhood residents. The confusion of these clinical and community roles in the community mental health center made life difficult in these centers, particularly for psychiatrists. This model calls on the psychiatrist to stay in role as a highly skilled technical expert with social and psychological expertise as well as medical skills. Much of the role strain of community psychiatry is eliminated in that the psychiatrist works in a stable medical institution that bridges into the neighborhood through the neighborhood-empowered community organization. The community staff are specialized social workers with skills to work outward in both directions.

It is important for the organizer to have an understanding of the life of a community—its community traditions, customs, values, and controls. The issue organizer who has a firm grasp and understanding of local traditions is able to organize with a rapidity and stability that is often astounding to observers. This is equally true of human service organizing; if the organizer has a good grasp on community life, his ability to gain legitimacy and acceptance by neighborhood residents will be enhanced. Equally important, the organizer must understand and respect medical intervention for the severely ill, unlike the old traditional organizer of the 1960s, who saw all symptoms as the product of environment and believed desperately ill schizophrenics and depressed patients could be cured with a touch of neighborhood support. Such social workers *cannot* link neighborhoods to effective care.

Part of an organizer's comprehension of the life of a community must be awareness of the specific agendas of local agencies and health care resources, as well as the constraints and dilemmas confronting those agencies. The organizer needs to communicate an appreciation of the expertise of professionals. Agencies, like community organizations, are best solicited to cooperate on the basis of self-interest. For an agency, this might include increased visibility, expanded community contacts, the attraction of more clients, and so forth. Most important, the organizer must escape from the guildism of any single profession (including one's own). The task of neighborhood empowerment is certainly not beating the drum for the glories of psychiatric social casework. In our experience, much of the distrust of community organizers in health professional circles stems from such self-serving guildism.

5. The empowerment model seems like a time-consuming and expensive process. Agencies need to see quick results, and they won't get them with this kind of approach. Also, isn't a "process" hard to replicate?

The process model does take considerable time to develop. There may not be quick, visible results. If a community mental health center or family service agency needs a quick "product," this approach won't satisfy those needs. In the long run, a process approach does prove to be cost effective. Large numbers of lay and professional helpers become involved in developing program initiatives that will be much more extensive than those that an agency's outreach workers could develop on their own. Much of the groundwork, in common with any good foundation, may be hard to see. Administrative staff need to be helped to realize that making a short-term investment in staff time now can result in impressive results over the long run.

In the implementation of the project, the pace of the work was especially critical in Milwaukee. There was initial distrust by Southside community leaders in the establishment of our project. Through the persistence and competency of organizer John Andreozzi, we were able to succeed. Professionals on the PAC tended to be too impatient. They tried to push things too fast. On a number of occasions, it was necessary to mediate conflicts arising because of pressure from the professionals conflicting with the desires of community leadership. Among our own staff, there was dynamic tension whether or not the process was moving fast enough. Why did it take three months before we could call our first meeting in Milwaukee? The Project Director regarded three months as a long time; the Field Organizer saw this as a short period. Such conflicts in our case were healthy—the field staff were challenged to justify their strategies, and the central office learned to respect the opinions and expertise of field staff who were closest to the community. Timetables were negotiated and renegotiated. We had the luxury, however, of four years to develop and test a model intervention. Those interested in developing similar neighborhood efforts must take care not to push too fast for results, lest they cripple the process as a result.

In numerous conference presentations about the project over the past four years, we found agency professionals most interested in "products," and only passingly interested in "process." They wanted to hear about self-help groups for widows, a community hotline, or a referral directory. They seemed uninterested in learning how development of these programs helped to empower community residents, to strengthen neighborhood helping networks, and to increase linkages between community and professional helping networks. Such thinking is understandable. People believe what they can see. A program is visible, a process much less so. Also, agency professionals are naturally most concerned about the problems (drugs, child abuse, separation/ divorce) and/or the population group (elderly, families, chronically mentally ill) that primarily relate to their own institution or agency. Administrators and others interested in trying to develop interventions similar to ours should realize that this tendency exists. Persistence is necessary to keep the focus on "process," rather than the simpler dividend or "product."

Many professionals we spoke to wanted a blueprint for replicating our work. There is no blueprint. We repeat that over and over. Although the goals of the model are universal, the strategies and methodologies need to be adapted to particular communities, taking into consideration questions of geography, race, class, age, sex, and ethnicity or neighborhood attachment.

> 6. Finding, building, and maintaining grassroots leadership is critical to any community organization effort; it seems especially difficult in this instance, when many people participate because of personal needs or problems. How is this obstacle surmounted?

Community leadership and leadership development is essential to any neighborhood-based organizing effort. A considerable amount of energy was expended by project staff in both cities in finding and developing organizational leaders. Though it was a time-consuming and difficult process, we have experienced considerable success. A brief description will help to highlight how we coped or didn't cope with some of our problems.

In Milwaukee there was difficulty focusing responsibility for the operation of the organization. The original SCO leaders were accustomed to being Board members, attending a few meetings, and having the staff follow through on Board actions, a traditional Board role. A community organization cannot survive or flourish this way. As new grassroots leadership began to emerge in SCO, this problem shifted to become an opportunity for leadership development. SCO staff had to concentrate on capacity building with newly involved people who, for the most part, were not established leaders.

There were three principal problems. First, many people who emerge from self-help groups are not willing or able to take on general leadership roles; they simply want to deal with their specific issues (i.e., widowhood or divorce). In every group, though, some natural leadership tends to emerge. Nurturance by staff encouraged these potential leaders to take responsibility for group functions. Staff then reduced their involvement to a consultative function. This capacity building process, that is, assisting people to develop the skills to lead groups and carry out projects, has been a major priority of the staff.

Secondly, in building a larger and more diversified SCO, new members were recruited for the Board in addition to the first leaders who already were overcommitted with various leadership roles. After the first year, SCO's Board grew to include more grassroots community residents who surfaced through participation in demonstration projects. It took some adjustment and trust-building to develop peer relationships between persons from these two different "social strata" in the community, the established leader and the grassroots resident. For example, having a nun as President of SCO during the second year was something of a new experience for members who grew up in a community where women did not typically occupy the top leadership posts.

Thirdly, most of SCO's grassroots leadership emerged from its self-help groups—widows, divorcees, agoraphobics, and so on. As a result, the identification of the leaders was primarily with their own self-help groups and only secondarily with SCO. Since none of these members were original members of SCO, they had difficulty identifying with any functions of SCO other than the enhancement of self-help. This led to problems in developing overall goals, objectives, and action plans, and in initiating new demonstration efforts.

Leadership development problems were different in Baltimore. Since this was already an established community organization whose governing board was largely representative of the community, one did not have to worry about issues of legitimacy. There could be direct development of a Task Force of natural helpers and other grassroots residents who were interested in mental health and human services. The success of our capacity-building process in creating a sense of community and enhancing the competency of Task Force members also led to one of the more serious problems. After an initial six-month organizing effort, the Task Force stabilized into a group of 20 residents who had a strong sense of esprit de corps. Attendance at meetings was very high. Participation in the group became an important component of these residents' social support system. Over time, the Task Force became a closed group. Although the Task Force members retained good ties to the rest of the community, they did not actively seek to enlarge their membership or participation.

On several occasions, project staff stressed the need for involving other residents as members of the group in order to infuse the group with fresh ideas and energy. Members were happy with the way that the group was functioning and resisted these changes. The group dynamics of closing boundaries in a support structure are well known. After a while, this led to a focus on maintaining existing projects rather than developing new ones. Although this tendency of "the group for its own sake" is common to many community organization efforts, had we realized earlier its ultimate impact on the course of the project, we could have focused the group's attention on their need for continuing membership renewal. With all our process emphasis, we overlooked a common danger in groups that focus more on support process than on outside tasks. This leads to consideration of the next issue.

7. The model requires a focus on process over product, but once products are organized—self-help groups, seminars, hotlines, and so forth—a lot of energy is needed for maintenance of these efforts. Is there enough energy left for continual involvement in process and new thrusts?

At the beginning of the projects, the energies of community groups in both cities were focused on analyzing community strengths and weaknesses, and developing intervention plans to address identified needs. The Task Forces, in effect, were starting with a clean slate, unhampered by the bureaucratic features of established organizations or the handicap of operational programs. Most of the interventive programs were established within 2 years. The grant called for continued development of new interventions and activities, but the community groups had been transformed from planning and oversight organizations into operations organizations. Staff had not given sufficient attention to the possibility of this happening and were unprepared to deal with it.

With the benefit of hindsight, we realize now that we should have established a planning or oversight committee in each city that would be charged with sustaining the process, continually measuring products against original expectations, in order to keep long-range project goals in sight. Alternatively, we might have separated planning and oversight from program operations by splitting the Task Force into subsections.

Of course, the process we have described occurs in any organization. One begins with ambitious goals. Then one finds that establishing and maintaining programs takes tremendous effort and significant organizational resources. Goals easily become displaced. Community mental health centers, for example, find themselves concentrating on whatever people come through the door for help, rather than on the extent to which the center is succeeding in meeting overall community needs.

In this model, it is critical that programs be evaluated from two perspectives. First, the program ought to be evaluated as to whether it is adequately meeting the needs of the target population for which it was conceived. In the case of our Hotline, the questions would be: "Are residents using it?" "Are they satisfied with the help they are getting?" Second, evaluations would see whether a specific program relates well to the process goals of the model. Does it strengthen the lay network? Does it create linkages between lay and professional networks?

Other problems in this project arose from our ambition to "institutionalize" a process. Once a community group or organization is created, once it develops programs and activities, it acquires a life of its own. Project staff were periodically torn between what activities/functions seemed best for the community groups and what was needed to meet the objectives of the grant. This conflict was most apparent in Milwaukee. Since there were no existing community organizations on the Southside, and SCO was developed from the beginning to fulfill the purposes of the grant, conflict would periodically ensue between the needs of building an organization, SCO, and the needs of the grant. All project staff were committed to leaving a solid foundation behind us when the project ended. To do this, considerable attention was devoted to the needs of SCO as an organization. Two years before the project ended, University of Southern California (USC) staff removed the SCO organizer from the USC payroll and gave additional funds to SCO itself to hire the same organizer directly. This move was intended to increase SCO's independence, but it also decreased USC's control over the demonstration project in Milwaukee. The organizer's priorities understandably became solely identified with SCO, rather that with both SCO and USC. Despite the difficulties cited, however, many projects were developed, tested, and successfully maintained.

8. The model requires involvement and commitment from a wide range of lay and professional helping groups—clergy, physicians,

natural helpers, neighborhood leaders, pharmacists, human service and mental agency staff, and school personnel. Isn't such
expectation of involvement unrealistic?

We have described an ideal model that involves all the lay and
professional helping groups. In actual practice, it may indeed be impossible to involve all of these groups in any given community. Actual
experience in the field comfirms this.

In both cities, direct involvement of pharmacists and physicians
was limited to research interviews. To interview these groups at all,
interview time was cut from 60 to 30 minutes. Both groups consisted
largely of private practitioners, whose time is expensive and filled with
obligations. We had minimal success in involving private physicians
and pharmacists in demonstration activities. This was a significant
problem. Our research findings show that the decision to seek professional help for psychological problems is heavily influenced by the recommendations of the residents' physicians. We developed plans to
work through the continuing education departments of medical schools
in the target area to offer a course for physicians on neighborhood support systems, but we never were able to follow up on this idea.

In both cities, there was extensive involvement with natural helpers, neighborhood leaders, and a wide array of human service and
mental health agency professionals. Involvement with the clergy varied
considerably in the two cities. In Baltimore, as we have seen, active
clergy involvement was maintained through a very successful series of
clergy/agency/community seminars and brown bag luncheons. In Milwaukee, the clergy provided a majority of the membership of SCO, the
early Board, and were crucial in assisting us to obtain both legitimacy
in the community and involvement by their parishioners. A successful,
well attended clergy/agency seminar was held in Milwaukee and followed up by 9 or 10 clergy/agency luncheons. They were difficult to
maintain, though, because clergy have so many meetings and commit-
ments. The project staff tried to get clergy to take staffing responsibility
for future luncheons, as clergy did in Baltimore, but this failed to occur.
As a result, contact with clergy has been limited to encounters on a one-
to-one basis with project staff. Ongoing linkages between clergy and
other helpers in Milwaukee did not develop as much as we hoped.

There are many groups in both cities with which we hardly worked
at all—the schools, the police, small businesses or labor unions, for
example. All these represent exciting opportunities for future partnership building.

9. Will this model work in all communities?

This model was designed for white, ethnic, working-class communities. It is a process model, and as such it is adaptable to other types of communities as well. Before discussing its application in different types of communities, we must stress our conviction that each and every community is unique. The model, as we have repeatedly said, cannot be used as a blueprint. The Baltimore and Milwaukee communities are both white, ethnic, working-class areas; yet they have key differences as well as great similarities. We varied strategies in implementing the model in each city. At the risk of being repetitious, we feel it important to highlight those similarities and differences here.

The Baltimore and Milwaukee neighborhoods are both principally stable, white, ethnic communities in which churches and ethnic and fraternal organizations are important and strong. Both communities are experiencing increasing problems of family stress and crisis, and neither has provided any organized support to the many separated/divorced or widowed individuals among them.

But significant differences also characterize the two communities. The Milwaukee community is predominantly composed of a single ethnic group—Polish. The neighborhood must be described as cohesive, informally organized, and rejecting of outside penetration. No organization represents the entire geographic area, neither are there block clubs nor improvement associations. Subparts of the area do not have commonly agreed on names. Thus, the identification of residents is with the Southside as a whole, or with a neighborhood park or church. The Baltimore community, on the other hand, is a mixed ethnic community whose boundaries are more open; it has a significant experience and history of participation in community organization activities. There are many block clubs and community improvement associations in South East Baltimore. Residents' identification is with the South East as a whole, and also with their particular area—Canton, Highlandtown, North of the Park, and so on.

The nature of the Southside Milwaukee community made the organizing process difficult. There have been few successful community organizing efforts in the target area. Many people belong to church, civic, and fraternal groups. There are many facets to this type of community organization. Individual churches of the same denomination maintain distinct identities; Roman Catholic parishes usually avoid mixing with Polish National Catholic and Eastern Orthodox parishes; Lutheran congregations are divided into various synods. Ethnic boundaries are evident among civic, fraternal, and veterans' groups. In addition to the splintering effect of these long-established institutions and organizations, community residents, especially among middle-aged and senior residents, have strong respect for established, traditional authority. This makes new organizations suspect by definition. These factors complicated the initial organizing of SCO and some of its pilot projects. The idea of a broad coalition working on a research and demonstration project in mental health, sponsored by a Pacific coast university, with a center based in Washington, D.C., in alliance with a medical college, and using federal funds, did not by any means win immediate acceptance. It was sometimes quite a task to explain to any audience what USC's Washington Public Affairs Center was doing in the Southside of Milwaukee!

The differences between the communities led to different organizing strategies. In Milwaukee, we initially focused on building an organization of established leadership—clergy, ethnic clubs, banks, agencies—while in Baltimore, we began to build and develop new and indigenous leadership for the Task Force. These differences led in turn to differences in role perceptions by the groups in each city. SCO Board members saw themselves providing leadership and endorsement, as indeed they were requested. Later adjustments had to be made to solicit involvement in the "nitty-gritty" project activities; the Baltimore Task Force represented the "doers" who were involved in day-to-day activities. Working on committees was part of the support system for many of the Task Force members. They enjoyed the process at the meetings and did not mind long or frequent meetings. Over time, however, the two groups became more similar as the membership of the SCO Board expanded to include residents who had become active in developing particular demonstration projects (the SCO Board included representation from each of the self-help groups and working committees).

Although the process of the model and its six objectives were the same in both cities, we have seen how implementation, even into reasonably similar communities, turned out to be different.

Return to the question of implementation in other communities— rural, nonwhite, or poor, for example. We can begin by observing that informal helping networks exist in every type of community—urban or rural; white, black, or Hispanic; poor, working-class, or middle-class. The problems of fragmentation and underutilization of services, lack of accessibility, and lack of accountability of services are also universal. We feel that the model process can apply to all communities, but that organizing strategies would have to be considerably different. For rural areas, the concept of neighborhood may be irrelevant, but visiting nurses play a much more significant helping role than they would tend to do in urban areas. Similarly, in Hispanic communities the spiritualist may represent a key natural helping resource unknown in white communities. The level of involvement of helpers and leaders called for in our model may seem unrealistic or unworkable in areas of high mobility or high levels of poverty. In the latter, survival concerns may dictate other priorities. Also, in high-income communities in which the residents purchase "private" instead of agency services, the model could not apply.

Just as we strongly criticize agency professionals for parachuting prepackaged services into the community, we do not see our model as a "package" to be used in its entirety in all communities. Rather, its objectives and processes can work in differing areas, with strategies adapted to the variations of community size, location, composition, helping networks, needs, and demographic and socioeconomic characteristics.

10. The model relies heavily on the neighborhood as a support system, yet for many persons, especially more mobile, upper-middle-class individuals, does the concept of neighborhood have real meaning?

It is certainly true that the concept of neighborhood is probably more significant to a working-class urban resident who has lived in the same area for 10 years, goes to church in his neighborhood, and belongs to ethnic, social, and fraternal organizations in his neighborhood, than it is to an upper-middle-class suburbanite who is more mobile and whose significant attachments—work, church, and organizational— tend not to be primarily neighborhood-based. Yet, programs and services are often geographically based, and the problems in the organization and delivery of these services can be an impetus for organizing people, even if their attachment to a place is not as strong as it is in urban, ethnic neighborhoods. To the extent that residents of a community purchase private services to meet their human service and mental health needs, then this model requires revision. It will be largely impractical and impossible to coordinate private caregivers who are independent entrepreneurs. But even in upper-middle-class, suburban communities, many residents do use public sector services, which tend to be just as fragmented as those in working-class urban areas. Moreover, the needs for indigenous support structures are no less select among the affluent. The model can be adapted for this population group, but it obviously will take very different forms. There will probably be more emphasis on organizing self-help groups and educational programs and developing interventions outside as well as within the community.

11. Support systems are not static; in fact, they undergo rapid changes. What are the implications of this change for the model?

We foresee three areas of significant change for support systems in the future—the role of ethnicity, the increasing number of women in the workplace, and the shift in population from central city to metropolitan area.

Ethnicity is not perceived only as the language and customs of other countries. Rather, it is a complex mixture of Americanized versions of European customs, working-class values, memories and "scars" from a not-too-distant minority-group status, a reaction to the "respectable" bigotry of people higher up in the "social order," and various other factors. Despite the recent upsurge of attention to ethnicity by scholars and the celebrated proclamation of a "new" ethnicity in our project cities, ethnicity apparently weakens with each passing generation. The grandchildren of Polish immigrants on the Southside of Milwaukee or of Italian immigrants in South East Baltimore still, at times, seek to escape their ethnic roots. Parents raised in a traditional ethnic working-class atmosphere experience difficulty relating to the mores of their teenage children, who are experimenting with drugs, new sexual attitudes, long hair, and jeans. In many families, both parents must work outside of the home for economic survival. The number of divorced and never-married parents has grown dramatically in ethnic communities, as elsewhere. These developments are not easily handled by the traditional family, church, or neighborhood networks, and the projects developed by SCO and SECO represent efforts to create new helping networks. For white ethnics, the most appropriate path to strengthened support systems may be in efforts to preserve the best aspects of their heritage and to mesh these with new practices that ensure the survival of their family and neighborhoods.

The research in Baltimore and Milwaukee found that a majority of the natural helpers in each community were women who did not work outside the home and who had been helping their neighbors, family, and friends for years. With a large increase in the number of women in the workplace over the past decade, the pool of potential helpers in the neighborhood may decrease dramatically in the future. There may be need therefore for more organized forms of informal help, such as the self-help groups and community hotlines developed through our model.

The neighborhood's importance as a support system varies among population groups. Communities such as the two study areas, where most of the informal help is now provided within a neighborhood context, can expect to experience a widening arena for help-seeking as more women join the work force. There is already evidence that the increasing number of women in management positions may make it easier for men to turn to co-workers (male as well as female) for support and assistance at times of crisis in their lives (Plaut, 1982). One can logically expect the workplace to become a more significant locus of social support in the future.

A major demographic change over the past decade has been a loss of population by shrinking urban centers to wider metropolitan areas, which have been growing in size. This has a number of implications. There has been an increase in elderly persons living alone and an increase in geographic distance between elderly persons and their children. Larger numbers of elderly persons are also moving into suburban areas. Support systems may have to become more geographically dispersed. There may be need for more organized systems of informal support to complement and enhance unorganized natural help. Gelfand and Gelfand (1982) suggest that for the elderly, the multipurpose senior center can serve an expanded role in providing opportunities for informal support systems to develop.

12. The model sounds like a rehash of the 1960s community action strategies. How is it different?

In actuality, the model differs in a number of significant aspects. First, the "war on poverty" bypassed conventional service providers, perceiving them as uninterested in or unable to serve the poor. Our model has stressed partnerships with existing service providers.

Second, the poverty program assumed that every community needed a community action agency with a set of prepackaged, nationally designed intervention programs. The focus was more on program than on process. Our model puts emphasis on process over program and recognizes that different program approaches and strategies are needed in different areas.

Third, the poverty program coopted many informal community leaders by offering them paid jobs at poverty agencies. Our model emphasizes strengthening the informal and formal systems, and recognizes the value of keeping the two systems separate though mutually interdependent.

Fourth, the poverty program underestimated the need for capacity building by community residents. Many residents on local boards were "run over" by professionals. We provided significant training, technical assistance, and resources to community residents before we brought them together with professionals.

Lest our comparison seem like an indictment of the "war on poverty," we should add that we think the poverty program made signifi-

cant accomplishments, including the provision of employment opportunities for the poor, the development of the beginnings of a political
base for black public officials, and the development and testing of strategies for community organizing and empowerment. Each of us was
involved in the poverty program in different ways, and our own work
since then has been positively influenced by our experiences.

CHAPTER 13

A Direction for the Next Decade

The empowerment of the voluntary and community sectors and the disencumberment of large, complex health institutions from clumsy government operation are the two principal issues confronting us in the field of mental health in the 1980s.

The conventional wisdom of recent years has portrayed health institutions and key informal support structures—such as families, communities, and religious institutions—locked in a "necessary" or "inevitable" conflict. The "pop" populism of these eras seemed to offer government regulation, control, and program evaluation as a panacea for improving mental health and treating mental illness. Our work suggests a radically different approach: a shift to greater power and autonomy for the richly variegated mosaic of American neighborhoods, combined with a system of excellent, high-technology mental health institutions.

The role of government in the field of mental health urgently requires redefinition. All levels of government have performed poorly in the ownership and direct operation of medical institutions. Governments have also performed poorly at all levels when authority has been entirely removed from neighborhood-based institutions. Ironically, the closer the level of government to the locality, the worse its performance seems to become in the delivery of care. The Veterans Administration system of psychiatric care has operated at a level far superior to the state hospitals which, in turn, have rarely sunk to the depths of some county and local asylums. Moving taxpayer investments from the federal institutes to the local governments releases neither the high-technology hospital nor the grassroots neighborhood structure from the wasteful ineptitude of government operation.

The kind of negative judgment that we and others have made contains no solutions for our predicament in and of itself. We hope that it will provoke enough new thinking to liberate us from the inertia of current dogma. At best, it may liberate enough energy and funds to enable us to address our problems more imaginatively.

Thus we have tried to demonstrate a process through which individual neighborhoods may begin to cope with their own mental health issues; through which the family, the church, the natural helping networks, the primary care physicians, the neighborhood leaders—in other words, the social networks that are the fabric of American community life—might deal with the problems of the "worried well," and provide the support structures necessary for those ill individuals who have the potential to return to their homes.

We propose a process blueprint, not a panacea; a direction, not a set of marching orders; an organized set of principles, not a regulation book. This blueprint strives to reduce the tension between high-technology institutions and neighborhood structures. Our approach is not to erase or blur the boundary between them, but to emphasize what each does best. Curable severe illness deserves the best that modern medicine can provide. Slovenly care will invariably produce disabilities that invariably prove far more expensive to all of us than early, effective intervention. Such high-quality care requires well-trained professionals.

But these same professionals cannot create neighborhood support structures—that is not their field of expertise. Similarly, those who have the know-how to set in motion the empowerment process in neighborhoods rarely manifest the same set of skills required to manage a severe disease such as acute, nonprocess schizophrenia. In our model, this boundary line is drawn between the Professional Advisory Committee and the Neighborhood Task Force.

Professionals in psychiatry, psychology, psychiatric social work, and psychiatric nursing are expected to operate within their professional capacities and are entitled to appropriate status, dignity, and respect. Similarly, neighborhood leaders, natural helpers, and members of other mediating structures in neighborhoods (such as the church) are entitled to meet with health professionals on a level of comparable status, dignity, and respect.

Partnership means an end to "zero sum games" in which the acutely ill patient and the deinstitutionalized patient, both of whom require support structures, are forced to compete for the same money.

To implement these goals, we offer the following policy recommendations:

Policy Recommendation 1

Community mental health must be redefined into specific neighborhood empowerment interventions and the fostering of genuine neighborhood structures, which can enhance mental health and offer support to those who are partially impaired.

Policy Recommendation 2

Care of the acutely ill who have remedial severe disorders belongs in specialized, high-technology institutions or their outreach clinics. The institutions must retain a clear but permeable boundary with neighborhoods.

Policy Recommendation 3

Direct funding should be earmarked for dissemination to neighborhood structures..

Policy Recommendation 4

Private contributions to defined neighborhood organizations, block organizations, self-help groups, and so forth, should count as full tax credits, up to a set amount.

Policy Recommendation 5

A National Endowment for Neighborhood and Communitities Organization (NENCO) should be established, with private contributions matched 50:50 by federal contributions.

Recommendations 3, 4, and 5 would facilitate a flow of funds to neighborhood structures that are not dominated by government. The investment tax credit is modeled after the precedent that has spurred capital renewal of industry. Renewal of key neighborhood structures ought to be a high national priority. We believe that investment in neighborhoods can renew the spiritual "capital foundation" of this nation. As the proposed national endowment would grow through a private/government partnership, interest might be used to fund new programs, new organizations, and new demonstration projects. Stimulating private contributions would help to ensure that government's role would diminish further as time goes on.

Policy Recommendation 6

Any fully accredited private, nonprofit, psychiatric facility treating any individual with a defined, treatable, severe psychiatric illness should, by law, receive the same reimbursement from that individual's private health insurance carrier as would be received by a general hospital for a physical illness.

There is a corollary to these recommendations:

Policy Recommendation 7

Mental health policy and model building should not be based primarily on dollar flow or on the economics of attrition.

The economics of attrition are just as likely to nurture survival of the *fattest* as survival of the *fittest*. State legislatures are currently being pressured by powerful constituencies to rescue the civil service at the expense of patient care. The current ambience seems to us to be creating a state snakepit. Neighborhood structures only rarely organize as effective political pressure groups. The questions thus arise: Who shall speak for the neighborhood? Who shall speak for the family? Who shall speak for the "worried well," for the institutionalized patient, and for those who lead lives of quiet despair?

None of us live so idyllically as to possess a guarantee that our households shall never know stress, anxiety, despondency, strife, or discord. None of us can be assured that our children are permanently immune to the drug epidemic or to severe adjustment problems. None of us can say with certainty that our current satisfactions in life will continue unmarred by the death or severe disability of the people we care about.

Tomorrow, any of us may urgently need social support through times of trouble, or health insurance to pay for skilled psychiatric help. Can we wait for tomorrow? Or have we the wherewithal to pursue these crucial concerns with as much persistence as the gun lobby or the oil lobby? Other vested interests are making sure that the available dollars are being diverted to support their priorities. Only too late do most of us concerned with mental health discover that the resources we need have been starved, and that the sole option available is that grotesque nineteenth century fossil, the government insane asylum. How many of us are willing to recognize that more than two-thirds of America's psychiatric beds are still located in such institutions?

Policy Recommendation 8

Federal, state, and local government should join the private sector in fostering and developing neighborhood and community support structures for the "worried well," the lonely, the mildly anxious, those who need help with their teenagers, and so forth.

Policy Recommendation 9

The state and county hospitals must cease their "reinstitutionalization" programs—the shift from inspected government hospitals to unmonitored core-city boarding houses and marginal nursing homes.

Policy Recommendation 10

Neighborhood support structures must be developed to reintegrate chronic, "partly" impaired patients in supportive environments. Such programs need priority funding.

Policy Recommendation 11

Severe, "totally" impaired, chronic patients must be placed in safe, humane havens, run in a truly cost-efficient manner. Such patients must no longer be spun in revolving doors from institution to boarding house and back. Precise medical, psychiatric, psychological, and social diagnoses must distinguish between those patients who require "safe haven" and those who can be reintegrated into special neighborhood structures.

The four preceding recommendations address the positive role that neighborhoods can play in the care of mental illness, as demonstrated by the projects reported in this volume. Deinstitutionalization does not mean kicking patients out of one institution and shunting them off to another. This heartless, political "shell game" must be exposed and halted. The nursing home has failed as a successor to the state hospital. The motives that fostered their development were often raids on Medicare and Medicaid funds, not "neighborhood" or "community" care. Politicians who try to escape Title XVIII and Title XIX regulations with the supposed "deinstitutionalization" of patients into decayed boarding homes or new state snakepits should be subjected to the strongest possible political sanctions. Neighborhood "dumping" has been a cynical distortion of the concept of neighborhood empowerment and community-based care.

Policy Recommendation 12

Government policy must be directed towards supporting the natural character of neighborhoods, their pluralistic individuality, their distinct specialness and uniqueness. This is possible through social microanalysis and maximal understanding of neighborhood infrastructure.

Policies based on macroanalysis—lowest-common-denominator procrustean beds—have distorted and even destroyed American neighborhoods. Neighborhood programs cannot be concocted in a federal food blender.

Policy Recommendation 13

Neighborhood policies must be based on the efforts and perceptions of involved individuals living in the neighborhoods. This is the essential feature of neighborhood empowerment.

Programs requiring large-scale development and elaboration by a multitude of outside professionals, the implementation of complex policies, the composition of voluminous forms and reports, special consultants, and similar bureaucratic practices only serve to increase alienation. The programs described in this volume were developed with one full-time community organizer per neighborhood. Staff must not and need not overwhelm genuine citizen involvement in neighborhoods.

Policy Recommendation 14

The neighborhood ought to be viewed as an arena for genuine program integration, as a viable alternative to the endless lists of categorical programs that now fragment and dehumanize care.

Categorical programs in mental health and human services have resulted in a constant shift of funding with a concurrent pattern of shifting program criteria. The effect: fragmentation of services. Even neighborhood leadership groups with sufficient sophistication to pick their way through labyrinths of bureaucratic criteria and submit complicated grant applications are finding that the priorities are being rewritten without mercy from year to year. Neighborhoods are—or have the potential to be—loci in which many services can come together; where whole human beings and whole families can properly be identified as the focal point of programming. Bureaucracies and institutions must no longer command the center of concern. Individual human beings, who live in individual neighborhoods, must receive individual care on an appropriate human scale.

Policy Recommendation 15

Accessibility of mental health services must be redefined in terms of: (1) acceptable, nonstigmatizing community support structures for the "worried well"; (2) rapid intervention for acutely ill psychiatric patients whose conditions are potentially remediable through intensive psychiatric care; and (3) neighborhood acceptance of the chronic, partially-impaired patients through special neighborhood-based social structures.

Clarification of these distinctions will both diminish stigma and foster effective early case finding for those who need such help. The concept of psychological acceptability of services deserves at least as much emphasis in the 1980s as the idea of geographic accessibility received in the 1960s and 1970s. Proper insurance will do more for financial accessibility than government subvention, which first may permit all of an individual's assets to be seized.

Policy Recommendation 16

Accountability is best served by direct neighborhood involvement in neighborhood programs and by program evaluation criteria required for Joint Commission on Accreditation of Hospitals approval of high-technology institutions.

Accountability by government committee has largely been a myth. Finance committees too often become lost in fine budget details; mental health committees too often seek dramatic impact, which wins head-lines for some official seeking elective office. Government bodies rarely will take the time for sustained, knowledgeable study, which might yield *real* accountability. One of the reasons for the success of many of the Milwaukee projects we have described was that a public board such as this actually functioned, and an unusually able, elected official, Supervisor Gerald Engel, helped to create such a climate of accountability for at least enough time to demonstrate that it could be done.

Policy Recommendation 17

Public policy must foster equity in mental health services.

So long as the poor, the elderly, the residents of the inner-cities, and the members of minority groups are found routinely incarcerated

in government institutions, while the affluent, the young , and the sub-
urb dwellers may use insurance funds for care in private psychiatric
hospitals and general hospitals, there can be no pretense of equity. The
paradox is that government care often costs more, both per unit of service and per spell of illness. Striving for equity also requires that capacity building be emphasized for certain neighborhoods, so that the necessarily elaborated social support systems become available to all.

Policy Recommendation 18

Neighborhood capacity building must be a central thrust of public
policy.

We have defined capacity building in chapter 4 in terms of people,
needs, policy, problem identification, and acquisition of skills. Building
cooperative partnerships among voluntary networks, understanding
delivery systems, dealing with local neighborhood obstacles, building
infraorganizations of mediating structures—all these are components of
neighborhood capacity building.

The agenda for the last decades of this century must go beyond cost
cutting, attrition, and apology. "When the elders at the gate are without
vision, the city is lost." What is our vision? The generation before us
made possible the community mental health revolution through painstaking theory building and innovations in service delivery from World
War II through the mid-1970s. Have we no more to offer than carping
criticism, revisionism, and retreat? Here we have offered our view. It
is a view of thriving neighborhoods. It is a view of involved citizens. It
is a view of renewed health institutions. Preeminently, it is a view of
care for human beings on a human scale.

Appendix
Survey Instrument—Community Leader and Helper Survey

S.E.C.O. HUMAN SERVICES AGENCY QUESTIONNAIRE[1]

Name of Agency _____

Address of Agency _____

Phone Number of Agency _____

Name of Director of Agency _____

Name of Interviewee _____

Identification Number _____

Neighborhood: _____

Time Began: _____

Name of Interviewer: _____

I.D. No. _____   Date: _____

A. Agency Information (Agency Directors only)

1. What do *you* see as the purpose of this Agency? _____
_____

2. Can you briefly describe your Agency's programs and services? _____
_____

3. How long (years) has this Agency been in existence? _____

4. What is your catchment area (service boundaries)? _____
_____

[1]Separate survey instruments were used for each of the seven interview categories in this survey. However, 75% of the questions were the same for each interview schedule. There were only minor differences between the Baltimore and Milwaukee interview schedules. The Baltimore Human Service Agency Questionnaire is included for representation purposes. Additional instruments are available from the authors.

5. What percentage of your clients reside outside of this catchment area? _ %

6. What is the eligibility criteria for your services? _____
   _____

7. Are your services focused toward any specific population group?
   (a) _____ Yes   (b) _____ No
   If yes, please describe: _____

8. What are the locations of your present services and hours of operations of
   each? _____
   _____

9. Does your Agency charge any fees for services?
   (a) _____ Yes   (b) _____ No
   If yes, on what basis? _____

10. Can clients be served in an immediate, same day basis?
    (a) _____ Yes   (b) _____ No

11. How many clients can be served at any given time? _____

12. Do you currently have a waiting list for service?
    (a) _____ Yes   (b) _____ No
    If yes, how long is the average wait? _____

13. What are the principal sources of referrals to your Agency? _____

14. Now, we would like you to describe your Agency's clients. How many clients
    did you serve in FY '76?   (a) _____
    What percentage are *male*?   (b) _____ %
    What percentage are *female*?   (c) _____ %

15. [*Interviewer:* Hand Card D]
    Please look at Card D. In which age group are most of your clients?
    (a) _____ Under 21   (b) _____ 21–35   (c) _____ 36–49
    (d) _____ 50–64   (e) _____ Over 65

16. Again looking at Card D, in which marital category are most of your clients?
    (a) _____ Single   (b) _____ Married   (c) _____ Divorced
    (d) _____ Widowed

17. Are the majority of your clients members of ethnic groups?
    (a) _____ Yes   (b) _____ No
    Please describe the ethnic background of your clients: _____
    _____

18. Why do you think that your clients come to your Agency instead of going to
    other places? _____

19. What service statistics does your Agency keep? Please describe.
    [*Interviewer:* ask for copy of intake form.] _____

20. Of your Agency's staff involved in services to clients, what percentage have
    Bachelor's degrees or below?
    (a)————%
    Of this group, what percent live in the neighborhoods you serve?
    (b)————%
    Can you briefly describe their responsibilities? _____
    _____

21. Is your Agency a member of any neighborhood organizations, task forces, coalitions, or advisory committees in the neighborhoods you serve?
 (a) _____ Yes   (b) _____ No
 If yes, please describe: _____
22. Is there any involvement from the community you serve in your services?
 (a) _____ Yes   (b) _____ No
 If yes, please describe: _____
23. What are your principal sources of funding? What are the approximate percentages of each toward your total funding? _____
_____

24. Are there any programs/services that you would like to see your Agency offer, but that you presently cannot because of financial limitations?
 (a) _____ Yes   (b) _____ No
 If yes, please describe those programs/services: _____

B. Agency Information (Mental Health Agency Directors only)

25. To many people mental health services have come to mean almost anything. This can create many problems. What do you feel should be the limits of your Agency's mental health services? _____
_____

26. What are the three major problems most often presented by clients to this agency?
 (1) _____
 (2) _____
 (3) _____

C. Agency Information (Non-Mental Health Agency Directors only)

27. Does your agency have a working relationship with any mental health agencies in your service area?
 (a) _____ Yes   (b) _____ No
 Please describe: _____
28. What do you see as the role of mental health agencies in your service area?
_____
_____

D. Human Service Agency Staff Information (All Staff)

29. Sex: (a) _____ Male
           (b) _____ Female
30. What is your age? _____ Years
31. Where were you born? _____
32. Where was your father born? _____
33. Where was your mother born? _____

34. Do you consider yourself to be a member of an ethnic group?
    (a) _____ Yes   (b) _____ No
    If yes, which ethnic group? _____
35. Do you live in any of the neighborhoods served by your Agency?
    (a) _____ Yes   (b) _____ No
    If no, where do you live?
    (c) _____ Baltimore City   (d) _____ Baltimore County
    (e) _____ Carroll County   (f) _____ Howard County
    (g) _____ Harford County   (h) _____ Other
36. What is your position in this Agency? _____
    How long have you held this position? _____ Years
37. How long have you worked for this Agency? _____ Years
38. Can you briefly describe what you do at this Agency? _____
39. Have you worked for any other human service agencies which serve South East Baltimore City?
    (a) _____ Yes   (b) _____ No
    If yes, which one(s)? _____
40. Do you have any training/degrees in the human services?
    (a) _____ Yes   (b) _____ No
    Can you briefly describe that training/degree? _____

E. Neighborhood Issues (All Staff)

41. What neighborhoods are within the service boundaries of your Agency?
    (a) _____ Broadway   (e) _____ Fells Pt./West of Park
    (b) _____ Canton   (f) _____ Highlandtown
    (c) _____ Eastern Highlandtown   (g) _____ North of the Park
    (d) _____ East Baltimore   (h) _____ South East Baltimore
    (i) _____ Other (please specify): _____
42. How would you rate these neighborhoods as places to live? [*Interviewer:* Read responses.]
    (a) _____ Excellent   (b) _____ Good   (c) _____ Fair
    (d) _____ Poor   (e) _____ Don't know (f) _____ No opinion
    Why? _____
43. In many neighborhoods, there are individuals of diverse ethnic backgrounds. Do you think that this is true for these neighborhoods?
    (a) _____ Yes   (b) _____ No   (c) _____ Don't know
44. How knowledgeable do you feel that you are of the values and attitudes of the different ethnic groups in these neighborhoods? [*Interviewer:* Read response categories.]
    (a) _____ Very knowledgeable   (b) _____ Knowledgeable
    (c) _____ Somewhat knowledgeable   (d) _____ Very little knowledge
    (e) _____ Not knowledgeable at all
45. What do you think were the three most important community issues in these neighborhoods last year?
    (1) _____   (2) _____   (3)_____

46. Who were the three most active people from the neighborhood involved with these issues? Can you give us their names?

(1) _____   (2) _____   (3) _____

F. Needs and Services (All Staff)

We have been talking in the last several questions about community problems that generally affect a lot of people. Now, we would like to get some idea about what happens in the neighborhoods served by your Agency when an individual or family has a problem.

47. Let's start with teenagers, ages 13–20. What is the major problem facing teenagers in these neighborhoods?

(a) _____ No problem   (b) _____ Don't know   (c) _____ Unsure
(d) Major problem: _____

48. What do people do who have this problem. _____

49. Of those who go for help, where do they go? _____

50. Which individual, group, or organization in the neighborhood is most helpful in meeting this problem?

(a) Don't know   (b) _____ Unsure   (c) _____ No help provided
(d) Name of individual / group / organization: _____

51. Are there any others that are also helpful? [*Interviewer:* Hand Card A and check responses below.]

(a) _____ Family   (i) _____ Pharmacists
(b) _____ Friends / Neighbors   (j) _____ Fraternal Organizations
(c) _____ Clergy / Churches   (k) _____ Neighborhood Improve.
(d) _____ Doctors   Assn.
(e) _____ Ethnic Clubs   (l) _____ Political Organization
(f) _____ Federation (SECO)   (m) _____ Senior Citizen Groups
(g) _____ Block Clubs   (n) _____ Other (please specify):
(h) _____ P.T.A.'s   _____
                                           (o) _____ No others

52. Can you tell us which professional Agency or Service is most helpful in meeting this problem?

(a) _____ Don't know   (b) _____ Unsure   (c) _____ No help provided
(d) Name of Agency / Service: _____

53. Are there any others that are also helpful? [*Interviewer:* Hand Card B. If category b, c, d, e, f, l, m is mentioned, ask for a specific name of program if possible.]

(a) _____ Dept. of Social Services   (e) _____ Mental Health Clinic _
(b) _____ Religious agency _____   _____
        _____   (f) _____ Mental Hospital_____
(c) _____ Medical Clinic _____   _____
        _____   (g) _____ Private Physicians
(d) _____ Hospital Emergency   (h) _____ Police Dept.
            Room_____   (i) _____ City Recreation Dept.

(j) _____ Public / Private School   (n) _____ Other (specify):_____
(k) _____ Alcoholics Anonymous   _____
(l) _____ Alcoholic / Drug Program   (o) _____ No others
_____
(m) _____ Private Psychiatrist _____
_____

54. Are there any other problems of teenagers in the neighborhoods?
[*Interviewer:* Hand Card C.]
(a) _____ Marriage   (l) _____ Job Problem
(b) _____ Parent / Child   (m) _____ Care of Elderly Relative
(c) _____ Boredom   (n) _____ Financial
(d) _____ Loneliness   (o) _____ School / Learning
(e) _____ Emotional / Psychiatric   Problems
(f) _____ Homosexuality   (p) _____ School / Behavior
(g) _____ Health Problems   Problems
(h) _____ Drugs   (q) _____ Other (specify): _____
(i) _____ Drinking / Alcoholism   _____
(j) _____ Unemployment   (r) _____ No Other Problems
(k) _____ Retirement Problem

55. Now let's discuss families. What is the major problem facing families in
these neighborhoods?
(a) _____ No Problem   (b) _____ Don't Know   (c) _____ Unsure
(d) Major Problem: _____

56. What do people do who have this problem? _____

57. Of those who go for help, where do they go? _____

58. Which individual, group, or organization in the neighborhoods is most helpful
in meeting this problem?
(a) _____ Don't know   (b) _____ Unsure   (c) _____ No help
provided
(d) Name of individual / group / organization: _____

59. Are there any others that are also helpful? [*Interviewer:* Hand Card A and
check responses below.]
(a) _____ Family   (j) _____ Fraternal Organization
(b) _____ Friends / Neighbors   (k) _____ Neighborhood Improve.
(c) _____ Clergy / Churches   Assn.
(d) _____ Doctors   (l) _____ Political Organization
(e) _____ Ethnic Clubs   (m) _____ Senior Citizen Groups
(f) _____ Federation (SECO)   (n) _____ Other (specify): _____
(g) _____ Block Clubs   _____
(h) _____ P.T.A.'s   (o) _____ No Others
(i) _____ Pharmacists

60. Can you tell us which professional agency or service is most helpful in meeting this problem?
(a) _____ Don't Know   (b) _____ Unsure   (c) _____ No help
provided
(d) Name of agency / service: _____

61. Are there any others that are also helpful? [*Interviewer:* Hand Card B. If category b, c, d, e, f, l, m is mentioned, ask for a more specific name of program, if possible.]

(a) _____ Dept. of Social Services
(b) _____ Religious Agency _____
_____
(c) _____ Medical Clinic _____
_____
(d) _____ Hospital Emergency Room _____
_____
(e) _____ Mental Health Clinic ___
_____
(f) _____ Mental Hospital _____
_____

(g) _____ Private Physician
(h) _____ Police Dept.
(i) _____ City Recreation Dept.
(j) _____ Public/Private School
(k) _____ Alcoholics Anonymous
(l) _____ Alcohol/Drug Program
_____
(m) _____ Private Psychiatrist ___
_____
(n) _____ Other (specify): _____
_____
(o) _____ No others

62. Are there any other problems of families in the neighborhoods? [*Interviewer:* Hand Card C.]

(a) _____ Marriage
(b) _____ Parent/Child
(c) _____ Boredom
(d) _____ Loneliness
(e) _____ Emotional/Psychiatric
(f) _____ Homosexuality
(g) _____ Health Problems
(h) _____ Drugs
(i) _____ Drinking/Alcoholism
(j) _____ Unemployment

(k) _____ Retirement Problem
(l) _____ Job Problem
(m) _____ Care of Elderly Relative
(n) _____ Financial
(o) _____ School/Learning Problems
(p) _____ School/Behavior Problems
(q) _____ Other (specify) _____
(r) _____ No other problems

63. We are interested now in examining persons who are separated or divorced. What is the major problem facing people who are separated/divorced in these neighborhoods?

(a) _____ No Problem   (b) _____ Don't know   (c) _____ Unsure
(d) Major problem: _____

64. What do people do who have this problem? _____

65. Of those who go for help, where do they go? _____

66. Which individual, group, or organization in the neighborhoods is most helpful in meeting this problem?

(a) _____ Don't know   (b) _____ Unsure   (c) _____ No help provided
(d) Name of individual/group/organization: _____

67. Are there any others that are also helpful? [*Interviewer:* Hand Card A and check responses below.]

(a) _____ Family
(b) _____ Friends/Neighbors
(c) _____ Clergy/Churches
(d) _____ Doctors
(e) _____ Ethnic Clubs

(f) _____ Federation (SECO)
(g) _____ Block Clubs
(h) _____ P.T.A.'s
(i) _____ Pharmacists
(j) _____ Fraternal Organizations

(k) _____ Neighborhood Improve.   (n) _____ Other (specify): _____
         Assns.   _____
(l) _____ Political Organization   (o) _____ No others
(m) _____ Senior Citizen Groups

68. Can you tell us which professional agency or service is most helpful in meeting this problem?
    (a) _____ Don't know   (b)_____ Unsure   (c) _____ No   help provided
    (d) Name of agency / service: _____

69. Are there any others that are also helpful? [*Interviewer:* Hand Card B. If category b, c, d, e, f, l, m is mentioned, ask for a more specific name of program if possible.]
    (a) _____ Dept. of Social Services   (g) _____ Private Physician
    (b) _____ Religious Agency _____   (h) _____ Police Dept.
         _____   (i) _____ City Recreation Dept.
    (c) _____ Medical Clinic _____   (j) _____ Public / Private Schools
         _____   (k) _____ Alcoholics Anonymous
    (d) _____ Hospital Emergency   (l) _____ Alcohol / Drug Program
         Room _____   _____
         _____   (m) _____ Private Psychiatrist _____
    (e) _____ Mental Health Clinic _____   _____
         _____   (n) _____ Other (specify): _____
    (f) _____ Mental Hospital _____   _____
         _____   (o) _____ No others

70. Are there any other problems of divorced or separated people in the neighborhoods? [*Interviewer:* Hand Card C.]
    (a) _____ Marriage   (l) _____ Job Problem
    (b) _____ Parent / Child   (m) _____ Care of Elderly Relative
    (c) _____ Boredom   (n) _____ Financial
    (d) _____ Loneliness   (o) _____ School / Learning
    (e) _____ Emotional / Psychiatric   Problems
    (f) _____ Homosexuality   (p) _____ School / Behavior
    (g) _____ Health Problems   Problems
    (h) _____ Drugs   (q) _____ Other (specify): _____
    (i) _____ Drinking / Alcoholism   _____
    (j) _____ Unemployment   (r) _____ No other problems
    (k) _____ Retirement Problem

71. Finally, let's take a look at the elderly. What is the major problem facing the elderly in these neighborhoods?
    (a) _____ No problem   (b) _____ Don't know   (c) _____ Unsure
    (d) Major problem: _____

72. What do people do who have this problem? _____

73. Of those who go for help, where do they go? _____

74. Which individual group, or organization in the neighborhoods is most helpful in meeting this problem?

(a) _____ Don't know   (b) _____ Unsure   (c) _____ No help provided

(d) Name of individual / group / organization: _____

75. Are there any others that are also helpful? (Interviewer: Show Card A and check responses below.)

(a) _____ Family
(b) _____ Friends / Neighbors
(c) _____ Clergy / Churches
(d) _____ Doctors
(e) _____ Ethnic Clubs
(f) _____ Federation (SECO)
(g) _____ Block Clubs
(h) _____ P.T.A.'s
(i) _____ Pharmacists

(j) _____ Fraternal Organizations
(k) _____ Neighborhood Improve. Assn.
(l) _____ Political Organization
(m) _____ Senior Citizen Groups
(n) _____ Other (specify): _____
(o) _____ No others

76. Can you tell us which professional agency or service is most helpful in meeting this problem?

(a) _____ Don't know   (b) _____ Unsure   (c) _____ No help provided

(d) Name of agency / service: _____

77. Are there any others that are also helpful? [Interviewer: Hand Card B. If category b, c, d, e, f, l, m is mentioned, ask for a more specific name if possible.]

(a) _____ Dept. of Social Services
(b) _____ Religious Agency _____
_____
(c) _____ Medical Clinic _____
_____
(d) _____ Hospital Emergency Room _____
_____
(e) _____ Mental Health Clinic _____
_____
(f) _____ Mental Hospital _____
_____
(g) _____ Private Physician

(h) _____ Police Dept.
(i) _____ City Recreation Dept.
(j) _____ Public / Private School
(k) _____ Alcoholics Anonymous
(l) _____ Alcohol / Drug Program
_____
_____
(m) _____ Private Psychiatrist _____
_____
(n) _____ Other (specify): _____
_____
(o) _____ No others

78. Are there any other problems of the elderly in the neighborhoods? [Interviewer: Hand Card C.]

(a) _____ Marriage
(b) _____ Parent / Child
(c) _____ Boredom
(d) _____ Loneliness
(e) _____ Emotional / Psychiatric
(f) _____ Homosexuality
(g) _____ Health Problems
(h) _____ Drugs

(i) _____ Drinking / Alcoholism
(j) _____ Unemployment
(k) _____ Retirement Problem
(l) _____ Job Problem
(m) _____ Care of Elderly Relative
(n) _____ Financial
(o) _____ School / Learning Problems

(p) _____ School/Behavior Problems   (r) _____ No other problems
(q) _____ Other (specify): _____

---

79. Do you think that the problems of widows/widowers are any different from the problems of the elderly that we have been discussing?
(a) _____ Yes   (b) _____ No   (c) _____ Don't know
(d) If yes, please describe. [*Interviewer:* Probe how problems are different and see where widows/widowers would go for help for these problems.]

80. Are there any other people in the neighborhoods who have special problems that we have not discussed?
(a) _____ Yes   (b) _____ No   (c) _____ Don't know
If yes, please specify: _____

81. Do you think that any of the problems of the various groups we have been discussing occur more frequently with any particular ethnic group(s)?
(a) _____ Yes   (b) _____ No
If yes, which problems? Which ethnic groups? Please describe and give some examples. _____

82. Do you think that different ethnic groups go to different places for help when they have problems? [*Interviewer:* Read responses.]
(a) _____ Yes, absolutely
(b) _____ Pretty much so, but there is some overlapping
(c) _____ No, they all use the same services
(d) _____ Don't know
(e) If a or b [*Interviewer:* Ask for some examples.] _____

83. Do you think that individuals in the neighborhoods know where to go for help when they have problems?
(a) _____ Yes, all do   (c) _____ A majority don't
(b) _____ A majority do   (d) _____ No, none do

84. In the neighborhood, is there a personal problem which you often hear about for which there is insufficient help available to people?
(a) _____ Yes   (b) _____ No
(c) If yes, what is that problem? _____

85. Are there any reasons why people in the neighborhoods would not seek help when they have a personal problem?
(a) _____ Yes   (b) _____ No   (c) _____ Don't know
If yes, please explain: _____
What can be done to overcome these obstacles? _____

86. Do you feel that people in the neighborhoods attach a stigma to the term "mental health"?
(a) _____ Yes   (b) _____ No   (c) _____ Don't know
If yes, how strong is this stigma? [*Interviewer:* Read categories.]
(d) _____ Very strong   (e) _____ Strong   (f) _____ Moderate
(g) _____ Mild   (h) _____ Almost nonexistent

87. What do you see as the major causes of the problems that we have been discussing _____

G. Human Services Agency Staff Counseling Role (Nonmental Health Agencies Only)

88. In the course of your work, do individuals from the neighborhoods you serve ever talk with you about their personal problems?
   (a) _____ Yes   (b) _____ No
89. How many individuals come to you per month? _____
90. Are the majority of the individuals that come to you for help members of ethnic groups?
   (a) _____ Yes   (b) _____ No
   Please describe the ethnic background of the individuals that come to you for help. _____
91. Which three problems are presented most often? [*Interviewer:* Hand Card C.]

   (a) _____ Marriage
   (b) _____ Parent/Child
   (c) _____ Boredom
   (d) _____ Loneliness
   (e) _____ Emotional/Psychiatric
   (f) _____ Homosexuality
   (g) _____ Health Problems
   (h) _____ Drugs
   (i) _____ Drinking/Alcoholism
   (j) _____ Unemployment
   (k) _____ Retirement Problems

   (l) _____ Job Problems
   (m) _____ Care of Elderly Relative
   (n) _____ Financial
   (o) _____ School/Learning Problems
   (p) _____ School/Behavior Problems
   (q) _____ Other (specify): _____
   _____
   (r) _____ No other problems

92. Now, we would like you to describe the individuals that come to you for help. What percentage are *male?*   (a) _____ %
   What percentage are *female?*   (b) _____ %
93. [*Interviewer:* Hand Card D.] Please look at Card D. In which age group are most of the individuals who come to you?
   (a) _____ Under 21   (b) _____ 21–35   (c) _____ 36–49
   (d) _____ 50–64   (e) _____ Over 65
94. Again looking at Card D, in which marital category are most of the clients that come to you for help?
   (a) _____ Single   (b) _____ Married   (c) _____ Divorced
   (d) _____ Widowed
95. Why do you think individuals come to you with their problems instead of going to other places when they have problems? _____
96. What can you do to help these individuals? Can you give me some examples? _____
97. If you cannot provide help yourself, do you make referrals to neighborhood groups or professional agencies?
   (a) _____ Yes   (b) _____ No
   If yes, to which groups or agencies have you made referrals in the last year?
   _____

H. Vignettes (All Agencies—Non-Directors only)

Now we would like to talk about something else. We would like to get your views concerning some short descriptions of behavior of individuals. These are fictional. [*Interviewer:* Hand Card E.]

First, I'm thinking of a man—let's call him Frank—who is very suspicious; he doesn't trust anybody, and he's sure that everybody is against him. Sometimes he thinks people he sees on the street are talking about him or following him around. A couple of times, now, he has beaten up men who didn't even know him, because he thought that they were plotting against him. The other night, he began to curse his wife terribly; then he hit her and threatened to kill her, because he said, she was working against him too, just like everyone else.

98. Does Frank have a problem?
    (a) _____ Yes   (b) _____ No   (c) _____ Unsure
99. If yes, how severe is the problem? [*Interviewer:* Read response categories.]
    (a) _____ Extremely severe   (b) _____ Severe   (c) _____ Moderate
    (d) _____ Mild   (e) _____ Hardly a problem at all
100. If Frank were a relative of yours, from what person would you first seek advice or opinions? _____
101. In your opinion, who could help Frank the most? _____
[*Interviewer:* Hand Card F.]

Here's a different sort of girl—let's call her Mary. She is happy and cheerful; she's pretty, has a good enough job, and is engaged to marry a nice young man. She has loads of friends; everybody likes her, and she's always busy and active. However, she just can't leave the house without going back again just to make sure she locked the door. And one other thing about her, she's afraid to ride up and down in elevators; she just won't go anyplace where she has to ride in an elevator to get there.

102. Does Mary have a problem?
    (a) _____ Yes   (b) _____ No   (c) _____ Unsure
103. If yes, how severe is this problem? [*Interviewer:* Read response categories.]
    (a) _____ Extremely severe   (b) _____ Severe   (c) _____ Moderate
    (d) _____ Mild   (e) _____ Hardly a problem at all
104. If Mary were a relative of yours, from what person would you first seek advice or opinions? _____
105. In your opinion, who could help Mary the most? _____
[*Interviewer:* Hand Card G.]

Now, I'd like to describe a 12-year-old boy—Bobby. He's bright enough and in good health, and he comes from a comfortable home. But his father and mother have found out that he's been telling lies for a long time now. He's been stealing things from stores, and taking money from his mother's purse, and he has been playing truant, staying away from school whenever he can. His parents are very upset about the way he acts, but he pays no attention to them.

106. Does Bobby have a problem?

   (a) _____ Yes   (b) _____ No   (c) _____ Unsure

107. If yes, how severe is the problem? [*Interviewer:* Read response categories.]

   (a) _____ Extremely severe   (b) _____ Severe   (c) _____ Moderate
   (d) _____ Mild   (e) _____ Hardly any problem at all

108. If Bobby were a relative of yours, from what person would you first seek advice or opinions? _____

109. In your opinion, who could help Bobby the most? _____

[*Interviewer:* Hand Card H.]

What about Bill? He never seems to be able to hold a job very long because he drinks so much. Whenever he has money in his pocket, he goes on a spree; he stays out 'till all hours drinking and never seems to care what happens to his wife and children. Sometimes he feels very bad about the way he treats his family; he begs his wife to forgive him and promises to stop drinking, but always goes off again.

110. Does Bill have a problem?

   (a) _____ Yes   (b) _____ No   (c) _____ Unsure

111. If yes, how severe is the problem? [*Interviewer:* Read response categories.]

   (a) _____ Extremely severe   (b) _____ Severe   (c) _____ Moderate
   (d) _____ Mild   (e) _____ Hardly any problem at all

112. If Bill were a relative of yours, from what person would you first seek advice or opinions? _____

113. In your opinion, who could help Bill the most? _____

I. Other Information Sources (114—All Staff; 115—Agency Directors only)

114. Very often in neighborhoods, there are people with no formal training in counseling whom people turn to when they are having problems. These individuals seem to be able to help people. Do you know of any people like this in your neighborhood?

   (a) _____ Yes   (b) _____ No

   If yes, can you give us the names and addresses of any of these individuals?

   _____

115. (Agency Directors Only) Can you give us the names of one or two members of the line staff of your Agency that you think would be helpful for us to interview? _____

Interviewer Comments: (Was interviewee responsive? Did s/he appear to answer based on knowledge/experience? Did s/he understand the questions in the interview? Please note any other comments.)

Time Interview Ended: _____

References

Agranoff, R. Services integration. In W. Anderson, B. Frieden, & M. Murphy (Eds.), *Managing human services.* Washington, D.C.: International City Management Association, 1977.

Ahlbrandt, R., Jr., & Cunningham, J. *A new public policy for neighborhood preservation.* New York: Praeger, 1979.

American Psychiatric Association. *A report of the American Psychiatric Association task force to develop a position statement on community mental health centers.* Washington, D.C.: APA, 1972.

Barrabe, P., & Von Mering, O. Ethnic variation in mental stress in families with psychotic children. *Social Problems,* 1953, 1, 18-53.

Benedek, E. *Training mental health professionals.* Paper prepared for the President's Commission on Mental Health, University of Michigan, 1977.

Berger, P., & Neuhaus, R. *To empower people: The role of mediating institutions.* Washington, D.C.: American Enterprise Institute for Public Policy Research, 1977.

Biegel, D. *Neighborhood support systems: People helping themselves.* Keynote Address, Pittsburgh Conference on Neighborhood Support Systems, Pittsburgh, Pa., 1979.

Biegel, D. *Help-seeking and receiving in urban ethnic neighborhoods.* Unpublished doctoral dissertation, University of Maryland, 1982.

Biegel, D., & Naparstek, A. Organizing for mental health: An empowerment model. *Journal of Alternative Human Services,* 1979, 5(3), 8-14.

Biegel, D., & Naparstek, A. The neighborhood and family services project: An empowerment model linking clergy, agency professionals, and community residents. In A. Jeger & R. Slotnik (Eds.), *Community mental health and behavioral-ecology: A handbook of theory, research, and practice.* New York: Plenum Press, 1982.

Biegel, D., & Sherman, W. Neighborhood capacity building and the ethnic aged. In D. Gelfand & A. Kutzik (Eds.) *Ethnicity and aging.* New York: Springer, 1979.

Bindman, A. Problems associated with community mental health programs. *Community Mental Health Journal,* 1966, 2(4), 333-338.

Bloom, B. *Community mental health, a general introduction.* Belmont, Calif.: Wadsworth, 1977.

Bowlby, J. The making and breaking of affectional bonds (Part 2). *British Journal of Psychiatry,* 1977, 130, 201-210.

Bradshaw, W. H. *Training psychiatrists for working with blacks in basic residency programs.* Paper presented at American Psychiatric Association Annual Meeting, Toronto, Canada, 1977.

Brandon, R. N. Differential use of mental health services: Social pathology or class victimization? In M. Guttentag & E. L. Struening (Eds.), *Handbook of evaluation research* (Vol. 2). Beverly Hills, Calif. Sage Publications, 1975.

211

Breton, R. Institutional completeness of ethnic communities and the personal relations of immigrants. *American Journal of Sociology*, 1964, *70*(2), 193–205.

Brown, B. Obstacles to treatment of blue collar workers, *New Dimensions in Mental Health*, June 1976, p. 5.

Butler, R. N. *Why survive? Being old in America.* New York: Harper & Row, 1975.

Butler, R. N. & Lewis, M. *Aging and mental health.* St. Louis: C. V. Mosby, 1977.

Caplan, G. *Support systems and community mental health.* New York: Behavioral Publications, 1974.

Caplan, G., & Grunebaum, H. Perspectives on primary prevention. *Archives of General Psychiatry*, 1967, *17*, 331–346.

Caplan, G., & Killilea, M. (Eds.). *Support systems and mutual help.* New York: Grune & Stratton, 1976.

Caplow, T., & Forman, R. Neighborhood interaction in a homogeneous community. *American Sociological Review*, 1950, *15*, 357–366.

Carter, J. Psychiatry's insensitivity to racism. *Psychiatric Opinion*, 1973, *10*, 21–25.

Cassel, J. Psychosocial processes and stress: Theoretical formulations. *International Journal of Health Services*, 1974, *4*, 471–482.

Clinebell, H. J., Jr. The local church's contribution to positive mental health. In H. J. Clinebell (Ed.), *Community mental health: The role of the church and temple.* Nashville: Abingdon, 1970.

Cohen, G. D. *Mental health and the elderly.* Unpublished issues paper. Rockville, Md.: National Institute of Mental Health, Center for Studies of the Mental Health of the Aging, 1977.

Collins, A. Natural delivery systems: Accessible sources of power for mental health. *American Journal of Orthopsychiatry*, 1973, *43*(1), 46–52.

Collins, A., & Pancoast, D. *Natural helping networks: A strategy for prevention.* Washington, D.C.: National Association of Social Workers, 1976.

Collins, A., & Pancoast, D. *Applying social work skills to natural networks.* Unpublished paper, 1977.

Congressional Budget Office, Congress of the United States. *Health differentials between white and nonwhite Americans.* Washington, D.C.: U.S. Government Printing Office, 1977.

Crocetti, G., Spiro, H. R., & Siassi, I. *Contemporary attitudes toward mental illness.* Pittsburgh: University of Pittsburgh Press, 1974.

Cumming, E., & Harrington, C. Clergyman as counselor. *American Journal of Sociology*, 1963, *69*, 234–243.

Cunningham, J. *The resurgent neighborhood.* Notre Dame, Ind.: Fides, 1965.

Cutright, W. *Racism, white flight and the changing neighborhood.* Paper presented at the 52nd Meeting of South Western Sociological Association, 1977.

Davidson, V. *Sex role stereotyping and diagnostic inequality.* Paper prepared for President's Commission on Mental Health, Department of Psychiatry, Baylor University, Houston, 1977.

Dennis, S., & Geruson, R. *Linking sociological and economic analyses of neighborhood change.* Paper presented at the Pennsylvania Sociological Society, Philadelphia, 1977.

Dohrenwend, B., & Dohrenwend, B. *Social status and psychological disorder: A causal inquiry.* New York: Wiley, 1976.

Doughton, M. J. *People power.* Bethlehem, Pa.: Media America, 1976.

Downs, A. *Understanding neighborhoods.* Washington, D.C.: Brookings Institution, in press.

Fandetti, D., & Gelfand, D. Attitudes toward symptoms and services in the ethnic family and neighborhood. *American Journal of Orthopsychiatry*, 1978, *48*(3), 477–486.

Gartner, A., & Reissman, F. *Self-help in the human services*. San Francisco: Jossey Bass, 1977.

Gelfond, D. & Gelfond, J. Senior citizen centers and social support. In D. Biegel & A. Naparstek (Eds.), *Community support systems: Practice, policy, and research*.New York: Springer, 1982.

Gilbert, N. Assessing service delivery methods: Some unsettled questions. *Welfare in Review*, 1973, *10*, 25.

Giordano, J. *Ethnicity and mental health*. New York: American Jewish Committee, 1973.

Giordano, J., & Giordano, G. Ethnicity and community mental health. *Community Mental Health Review*, Summer 1976.

Glazer, N. The limits of social policy. *Commentary*, 1971, *52*,(3), 51–58.

Gordon, J. S. New roads to mental health. *Washington Post*, February 13, 1977.

Greer, S. Neighborhood. *International encyclopedia of the social sciences*, (Vol. 2). New York: Crowell, Collier, & MacMillan, 1968.

Grier, W., & Cobbs, P. *Black rage*. New York: Basic Books, 1968.

Gurin, G., Veroff, J., & Feld, S. *Americans view their mental health*. New York: Basic Books, 1960.

Gussow, Z., & Tracy, G. S. The role of self-help clubs in adaptation to chronic illness and disability. *Social Science and Medicine*, 1976, *10*, 407–414.

Guttentag, M., Salasin, S., Legge, W. W., & Bray, H. *Sex differences in the utilization of publicly supported mental health facilities: The puzzle of depression*. Rockville, MD.: Mental Health Services, National Institute of Mental Health, 1976.

Hallman, H. *Neighborhood government in a metropolitan setting*. Beverly Hills: Sage Publications, 1974.

Halroyd, J. C., & Brodsky, A. M. Psychologists' attitudes and practices regarding erotic and nonerotic physical contact with patients. *American Psychologist*, 1977, *32*, 843–849.

Hamburg, B., & Killilea, M. Relation of social support, stress, illness and use of health services. *U.S. surgeon general's report: Background papers*. Washington, D.C.: Government Printing Office, 1979.

Haugk, K. Unique contributions of churches and clergy to community mental health. *Community Mental Health Journal*, 1976, *12*(1), 20–28.

Hojnacki, W. P. What is a neighborhood? *Social Policy*, 1979, *10*(2), 47–52.

Hollingshead, A., & Redlich, F. *Social class and mental illness, a community study*. New York: Wiley, 1958.

Jacquet, C. H., Jr. (Ed.). *Yearbook of American churches, 1972*. Nashville: Abingdon, 1972.

Jacobs, J. *The death and life of great American cities*. New York: Vintage, 1961.

Joint Commission on Mental Illness and Health. *Action for mental health: Final report of the Joint Commission*. New York: Basic Books, 1961.

Kahn, A. *Service delivery at the neighborhood level: Experience theory and facts*. Presented at the Symposium on Neighborhood Service Delivery, Community Service Society of New York, October 1974.

Kardiner, S., Fuller, M., & Mensh, I. A survey of physicians' attitudes and practices regarding erotic and nonerotic contact with patients. *American Journal of Psychiatry*, 1973, *130*, 1077–1081.

Keller, S. *The urban neighborhood: A sociological perspective*. New York: Random House, 1968.

Klein, D. The meaning of community in a preventive mental health program. *American Journal of Public Health*, 1969, 59(11), 2005–2012.

Kotler, M. *Neighborhood government: The local foundation of political life*. Indianapolis: Bobbs-Merrill, 1969.

Kruger, D. *The relationship of ethnicity to utilization of community mental health centers*. Unpublished doctoral dissertation, University of Texas at Austin, 1974.

Larson, R. F. The clergyman's role in the therapeutic process: Disagreements between clergymen and psychiatrists. *Psychiatry*, 1968, *31*, 250–263.

Lee, N. H. *The search for an abortionist*. Chicago: University of Chicago Press, 1969.

Levy, P. Unloading the neighborhood bandwagon. *Social Policy*, 1979, *10*, 28–32.

Lewis, H. *Child rearing among low income families*. Washington, D.C.: Health and Welfare Council of the National Capitol Area, 1961.

Liebow, E. *Tally's corner*. Boston: Little, Brown, 1967.

Litwak, E. Voluntary associations and neighborhood cohesion. *American Sociological Review*, 1961, *26*(2), 258–271.

Litwak, E., & Szelenyi, I. Primary group structures and their functions: Kin, neighbors and friends. *American Sociological Review*, 1969, *34*, 465–481.

Lowi, T. *The end of liberalism*. New York: W. W. Norton, 1969.

Macias, R. F. U.S. Hispanics in 2000 A.D.—Projecting the number. *Agenda*, 1977, *7*(3), 16–20.

Mann, P. The neighborhood. In R. Guttman & D. Popenoe (Eds.), *Neighborhood, city and metropolis*. New York: Random House, 1970.

Maracek, J. Powerlessness and women's psychological disorders. Voices. *Journal of the American Academy of Psychotherapists*, 1976, *12*, 241.

Marris, P., & Rein, M. *Dilemmas of social reform*. New York: Atherton, 1969.

Martineau, W. H. Informal social ties among urban black Americans: Some new data and a review of the problems. *Journal of Black Studies*, 177, *8*, 83–104.

McCann, R. *The churches and mental health* (Monograph Series No. 8). New York: Basic Books, 1962.

McKinlay, J. Social networks, lay consultation and help seeking behavior. *Social Forces*, 1973, *51*(3), 275–292.

Mitchell, J. C. (Ed.). *Social networks in urban situations*. New York: Oxford University Press, 1969.

Morris, D., & Hess, K. *Neighborhood power: The new localism*. Boston: Beacon, 1975.

Miller, S. & Altschuler, A. *Services for people: Report of the Task Force on Organization of Social Services*. U.S. Department of Health, Education, and Welfare, February, 1968.

Moynihan, D. *The Negro family: The case for national action*. Washington, D.C.: U.S. Department of Labor, Office of Planning and Research, 1965.

Moynihan, D. *Perspective on poverty: On understanding poverty*. New York: Basic Books, 1968.

Mudd, J. *Beyond community control: A neighborhood strategy for city government*. Unpublished paper, Woodrow Wilson International Center for Scholars, Washington, D.C., 1976.

Mumford, L. *The urban prospect*. New York: Harcourt, 1968.

Myers, J., & Bean, L. *A decade later: A follow up of social class and mental illness*. New York: Wiley, 1968.

Naparstek, A. J. *A socio-historical overview of community action program social services: Assumptions and implications for social service policy*. Unpublished paper, Brandeis University, 1971.

Naparstek, A. J. *Public opinions toward the economic opportunity act: The impact on the working class.* Unpublished doctoral dissertation, Brandeis University, 1972.

Naparstek, A. J. *Policy options for neighborhood empowerment.* National Urban Policy Roundtable, 1976.

Naparstek, A. J., & Biegel, D. Partnership building in mental health and human services: A community support systems approach. Subcommittee on Health and the Environment, Committee on Interstate and Foreign Commerce, House of Representatives. *Community support for mental patients.* Washington, D.C.: U.S. Government Printing Office, 1979.

Naparstek, A. J., & Biegel, D. A policy framework for community support systems. In D. Biegel & A. Naparstek (Eds.), *Community support systems and mental health: Research, practice and policy.* New York: Springer, 1982.

Naparstek, A. J., & Biegel, D. Community support systems: An alternative approach to mental health service delivery. In U. Rueveni, R. Speck, & J. Speck (Eds.), *Therapeutic interventions: Healing strategies for human systems.* New York: Human Sciences Press, 1982.

Naparstek, A., & Haskell, C. Neighborhood approaches to mental health services. In L. Macht, D. Scherl, & S. Sharfstein (Eds.), *Neighborhood psychiatry.* Lexington, Ma.: Lexington Books, 1977.

Naparstek, A., & Haskell, C. Neighborhood approaches to urban capacity building in urban affairs papers: A symposium issue. In C. Newland (Ed.), *Urban capacity building* (Vol. 3). Blacksburg, VA.: Virginia Polytechnic Institute, 1981.

Naparstek, A., Biegel, D., & Spence, B. Community analysis data report, Volume 1: First level analysis *Catalog of Selected Documents in Psychology,* 1979, 1, 88–89. (Ms. No. 1964)

National Commission on Neighborhoods. Case Study. Appendix, Volumes 1 and 2. *Final report to the President and Congress of the United States.* Washington, D.C.: U.S. Government Printing Office, 1979. (a)

National Commission on Neighborhoods. *Final report to the President and Congress of the United States.* Washington, D.C.: U.S. Government Printing Office, 1979. (b)

National Conference on Social Welfare. *The future of social services in the United States.* Washington, D.C.: National Conference on Social Welfare 1977.

Neugarten, B. Age groups in American society and the rise of the young old. *The Annals,* 1974, *415,* 187–212.

O'Brien, D. *Neighborhood organization and interest group process.* Princeton: Princeton University Press, 1975.

Opler, M. *Culture and social psychiatry.* New York: Atherton, 1967.

Ostrom, V. *The intellectual crisis in American public administration.* Tuscaloosa: University of Alabama Press, 1973.

Padilla, A. M., & Ruiz, R. A. *Latino mental health: A review of the literature* (Department of Health, Education and Welfare Pub. No. (HSM) 73-9143). Washington, D.C.: U.S. Government Printing Office, 1973.

Padilla, A. M., Ruiz, R. A., & Alvarez, A. Community mental health services for the Spanish speaking/surnamed population. *American Psychologist,* 1975, *30,* 892–905.

Pancoast, D. *A method of assisting natural helping networks.* Unpublished paper, 1978.

Pargament, K. I. The interface among religion, religious support systems and mental health. In D. Biegel & A. Naparstek (Eds.), *Community support systems and mental health: Research, practice and policy.* New York: Springer, 1982.

Park, R. E. The city: Suggestions for the investigation of human behavior in the city environment. *American Journal of Sociology,* 1915, *10,* 517–612.

Perlman, J. Grassroots empowerment and government response. *Social Policy*, 1979, *10*, 16.

Plaut, T. Primary prevention in the 80's: The interface with community support systems. In D. Biegel & A. Naparstek (Eds.), *Community support systems and mental health: Practice, policy, and research.* New York: Springer, 1982.

President's Commission on Mental Health. *Report to the President* (Vols. 1–4). Washington, D.C.: U.S. Government Printing Office, 1978.

Radloff, L. Sex differences in depression: The effects of occupation and marital status. *Sex Roles: A Journal of Research*, 1975, *1*(3), 110–112.

Rainwater, L. Some aspects of lower class sexual behavior. *Journal of Social Issues*, 1966, *22*, 96–108.

Rainwater, L. *Making the good life: Working class, family and life style.* Unpublished manuscript, October 1970.

Rein, M. *Social policy.* New York: Random House, 1970.

Reissman, F. The "helper therapy" principle. *Social Work*, 1965, *10*, 27–32.

Rieff, R. Mental health manpower and institutional change. *American Psychologist*, 1966, *21*(6), 540–548.

Roos, J. L., & Broden, T. F. *Neighborhood conservation.* South Bend, Ind.: South Bend Observatory, 1976.

Rose, S. *Community action programs: The relationship between initial conception of the poverty problems, derived intervention, strategy, and program implementation.* Unpublished doctoral dissertation, Brandeis University, 1970.

Ryan, W. Emotional disorder as a social problem: Implications for mental health programs. *American Journal of Orthopsychiatry*, 1971, *41*(4), 645–683.

Sarason, S., et al. *Human services and resource networks.* San Francisco: Jossey Bass, 1977.

Schiff, S. Community accountability and mental health services. In D. B. Denner & R. Price (Eds.), *Community mental health: Social action and reaction.* New York: Holt, Rinehart & Winston, 1973.

Schumacher, E. F. *Small is beautiful: Economics as if people matter.* New York: Harper & Row, 1973.

Seidler-Feller, D. Process and power in couples psychotherapy: A feminist view. Voices. *Journal of the American Academy of Psychotherapists*, 1976, *12*, 5–8.

Sherman, W., & Haskell, C. *Capacity building monograph.* Unpublished, University of Southern California, 1980.

Shevsky, E., & Bell, W. *Social area analysis.* Stanford, Calif.: Stanford University Press, 1955.

Siassi, I., Crocetti, G., & Spiro, H. R. Psychiatry and social class. *Social Psychiatry*, 1976, *11*, 99–105.

Silverman, P. R. The widow as a caregiver in a program of preventive intervention with other widows. *Mental Hygiene*, 1970, *54*, 540–547.

Silverman, P. R. Mutual help groups: A guide for mental health workers (Department of Health, Education and Welfare Pub. No. 78-646). Washington, D.C.: U.S. Government Printing Office, 1978.

Slater, P. *The pursuit of loneliness: American culture at the breaking point.* Boston: Beacon, 1970.

Smith, M. B., & Hobbs, N. The community and the community mental health center. *American Psychologist*, 1966, *21*, 499–509.

Smith, S., & Collins, A. *Training professionals to work with natural networks.* Unpublished paper, 1979.

Solis, A. *Utilization of community mental health services by the Spanish surname populations in California counties with 5 percent or more Spanish surnamed population 1976–1977.* Paper presented at the Working Conference on the Political and Economic Status of Hispanic Community Mental Health Centers. University of California, Los Angeles: Spanish Speaking Mental Health Research Center, July 1977.

Spergel, I. A. (Ed.). *Community organization studies in constraint.* Beverly Hills: Sage Publications, 1972.

Spiegel, D. Self-help and mutual support groups: A synthesis of the recent literature. In D. Biegel & A. Naparstek (Eds.), *Community support systems and mental health: Practice, policy, and research.* New York: Springer, 1982.

Spiegel, H. *Citizen participation.* Washington D.C.: National Training Laboratory for Applied Behavioral Sciences, 1968.

Spiegel, J. Some cultural aspects of transference and counter transference. In M. W. Zald (Ed.), *Social welfare institutions.* New York: Wiley, 1965.

Spiro, H. R. On beyond mental health centers: A planning model for psychiatric care. *AMA Archives of General Psychiatry,* 1969, *21,* 646–655.

Spiro, H. R. *The future of the state hospital.* Presentation at the Institute of Hospital and Community Psychiatry, Boston, November 1980. (a)

Spiro, H. R. Prevention in psychiatry: Primary, secondary and tertiary. In H. Kaplan, A. H. Freedman, & B. J. Sadlock (Eds.), *Comprehensive textbook in psychiatry* (3rd ed.). Baltimore: Williams and Wilkins, 1980. (b)

Spiro, H. R. Crisis in inpatient services. In R. Hall (Ed.), *Crisis in American psychiatry.* New York: Plenum Press, 1982.

Spiro, H. R., Siassi, I., & Crocetti, G. Cost financed mental health facility, II: Utilization profile of a labor union program. *Journal of Nervous & Mental Disease,* 1975, *160,* 241–248. (a)

Spiro, H. R., Siassi, I., & Crocetti, G. Cost financed mental health facility, III: Economic issues and implications for future patterns of health care. *Journal of Nervous & Mental Disease,* 1975, *160,* 249–254. (b)

Spiro, H. R., Crocetti, G., Siassi, I., Ward, R., & Hansen, E. Cost financed mental health facility, I: Clinical care patterns in labor union mental health program. *Journal of Nervous & Mental Disease,* 1975, *160,* 231–240.

Spurlock, J. *Mental health of women.* Paper prepared for President's Commission on Mental Health, 1977.

Srole, L., & Fisher, A. K. (Eds.). *Mental health in the metropolis: The midtown Manhattan study.* New York: McGraw Hill, 1960.

Sue, S., McKinney, H., Allen, D., & Hall, J. *Delivery of community mental health services to black and white clients.* Seattle: University of Washington, 1974.

Sundquist, J. *Politics and policy—the Eisenhower, Kennedy, and Johnson years.* Washington, D.C.: The Brookings Institution, 1968.

Thomas, A., & Sillen, S. *Racism and psychiatry.* New York: Brunner/Mazel, 1972.

Thomas, C. S., & Comer, J. P. Racism and mental health services. In C. Willie, B. M. Kramer, & B. Brown (Eds.), *Racism and mental health.* Pittsburgh: University of Pittsburgh Press, 1973.

Toennies, F. *Community and society* (C. P. Loomis, Ed. and trans.). East Lansing: Michigan State University Press, 1957. (Originally published 1887.)

Veroff, J., Douvan, E., & Kulka, R. *Americans view their mental health.* Ann Arbor: Survey Research Center, University of Michigan, 1976.

Warren, D. Neighborhood in urban areas. In J. Turner (Ed.), *The encyclopedia of social work.* New York: National Association of Social Workers, 1977.

Warren, D., & Clifford, D. *Help seeking behavior and the neighborhood context: Some preliminary findings on a study of helping networks in the urban community.* Unpublished paper, Program in Community Effectiveness, Institute of Labor and Industrial Relations, University of Michigan, 1975.

Warren, R. *The community in America.* Chicago: Rand McNally, 1963.

Warren, R. (Ed.). *New perspectives on the American community* (3rd ed.). Chicago: Rand McNally College Publishing, 1977.

Warren, R. B., & Warren, D. I. *The neighborhood organizer's handbook.* Notre Dame, Ind.: University of Notre Dame Press, 1977.

Washnis, G. *Municipal decentralization and neighborhood resources.* New York: Praeger, 1972.

Weissman, M. *Depressed women: Traditional and non traditional therapies.* Paper presented at the Eighth Annual Symposium, Effective Psychotherapy. Houston, Tx.: Texas Research Institute of Mental Sciences, November 1975.

Wilcox, P. Positive mental health in the black community: The black liberation movement. In C. V. Wille, B. M. Kramer, & B. S. Brown (Eds.), *Racism and mental health.* Pittsburgh: University of Pittsburgh Press, 1973.

Wilensky, H., & Lebeaux, C. *Industrial society and social welfare.* New York: The Free Press, 1965.

Winston, E. Public welfare. In H. Lusie (Ed.), *Encyclopedia of social work.* New York: National Association of Social Workers, 1965.

Woodson, R. *A summons to life.* Cambridge: Ballinger, 1981.

Yin, R., & Yates, D. *Street level governments: Assessing decentralization and urban services* (National Sciences Foundation Report T-1527). Santa Monica: Rand Corporation, 1974.

Zborowski, M. *People in pain.* San Francisco: Jossey Bass, 1964.

Zimmerman, J. *The federated city.* New York: St. Martins, 1972.

Index

AFDC (Aid to Families with Dependent Children), 42
Accessibility
  as factor in formation of
    neighborhood partners, 58, 195
Accountability
  as factor in mental health and human
    service delivery, 47, 50, 57–58, 195
Acute treatment hospitals, 6
Addams, Jane, 15
Adolescents
  resources for, 108
Aid to Families with Dependent
  Children (AFDC), 42
Alcoholics Anonymous, 80
Alienation
  and neighborhood, 19–30, 62
Alinsky, Saul, 15–16
American federalism, 14
American Indians
  mental health and, 72
  See also Racial minorities
Americans, Asian/Pacific
  mental health and, 72
  See also Racial minorities
Asylums, 31, 32

Baltimore, Md.
  action research in, 128–131
  application of Community
    Empowerment Model in, 50, 94,
    102, 117–135
  community described, 92, 117–119
  community leader and helper survey,
    105
  community obstacles, 113–115
  community potentials, 110–112, 115–
    116

Baltimore, Md. (*cont.*)
  community resident survey, 104–105
  demonstration programs, 131–134
  development and structure of
    Community Task Force, 121–126
  Professional Advisory Committee,
    126–128
  Professional mental health service
    system, 118
  Southeast Community Organization,
    102, 103, 119–120, 121–126
Barriers, economic, 6
Blacks
  institutionalization among, 71
  mental illness and, 70–71
Bureau of the Census, 41
Bureau of Labor Statistics, 41

CAP (Community Action Program), 42, 43
CMHC Act. *See* Community Mental
    Health Centers Act (1963)
Capacity building, 5, 196
Centralization
  of decision-making in cities, 15
  of service delivery systems, 12
Chronic social breakdown syndrome.
    See Gruenberg's syndrome
City
  as basis of life in gesellschaft, 21
  distribution of resources within, 15
Clergy
  role in community mental health, 77–
    80, 107, 111
Combat neuroses, 33
Community Action Program, 42, 43
Community Mental Health Centers Act
    (1963), 3, 33–34, 66